Moving and Handling of People in Care Settings

A Holistic and Compliance Manual Handling Training Guide

Clārĭtās®

2024

Moving & Handling of People in Care Settings

Claritas Publishing Limited is a strategic UK publisher.

Illustration & text copyright © 2024 by Claritas Publishing Limited
Text copyright © 2024 by A A Jude.

claritaspublishing.co.uk
info@claritaspublishing.co.uk
claritaspublishingltd@gmail.com
Registered Address: 27 Old Gloucester Street, London WC1N 3AX

ISBN 978-1-7384350-0-5

9 781738 435005 >

All rights reserved. It is illegal to reproduce, duplicate, or transmit any part of this document electronically or in mechanical forms such as photocopying, printing, recording or otherwise. All enquiries regarding any extracts or re-use of any material in this book should be addressed to the publishers, Claritas Publishing Limited.

Every effort has been made to ensure the accuracy of the contents of this manual. The Author / Editor or Claritas Publishing Ltd does not accept responsibility for any errors of fact or omission in this publication, and users should take appropriate professional advice before the moving and handling activity is implemented.

FIRST EDITION 2024 (Paperback)

A CIP catalogue record for this manual/book is available from the British Library: ISBN 978-1-7384350-0-5

ISBN 978-1-7384350-2-9 (hardback)
ISBN 978-1-7384350-1-2 (eBook)

Book classification: self-help; legal; health and social care; training; nursing; health and safety.

Claritas Health and Social Care Series

Moving & Handling of People in Care Settings

ACRONYMS & ABBREVIATIONS 8
GLOSSARY OF TERMS 10
ACKNOWLEDGEMENT 12
FOREWORD 13

CHAPTER ONE 14

INTRODUCTION 14

ABOUT THIS MANUAL 14
   Compliance with the law as a dilemma and solution 14
   Existing manuals, handbooks and guides 16
   Who should read this manual? 17
   The Manual's objectives 18
   The structure 19
SELECTED TERMS DEFINITIONS 20
   Employee 20
   Employer 21
   Lifting equipment 21
   Lifting operation 22
   Load 22
   Manual handling operations 22
AN OVERVIEW OF STAKEHOLDERS IN MOVING AND HANDLING 22
   The individual or service user 22
   The carer and the care worker 23
   The employer/organisation 26
   Trainers 28
   Significant Others 28

CHAPTER TWO 30

THE LEGISLATION 30

UNDERSTANDING MANUAL HANDLING AND MOVING AND HANDLING OF PEOPLE 30
   Manual handling and moving and handling 30
   The general purposes of relevant legislation 31
LEGISLATION IN MOVING AND HANDLING 32
   MHOR 1992 / 2002 32
   LOLER 1998 34
   PUWER 1998 35

Moving & Handling of People in Care Settings

MHSWR 1999 36
HSWA 1974 37
RIDDOR 2013.. 38
Care Act 2014... 40
OTHER LEGAL AND COMPLIANCE ISSUES IN MOVING AND HANDLING 41
Duty of care as a legal obligation 41
Care plan (and handling plan)... 41
Policy and procedure.. 43
Ergonomic risk assessment process in moving and handling................ 43
Abuse 45
Consent 48
Deprived liberties 48
Mental Capacity Act 2005... 49
Work ethics 50
Emergency care and first aid 51
GDPR 2018 (DPA)... 51
Domiciliary and care home contexts 52

CHAPTER THREE **53**

HOLISTIC APPROACH TO MOVING AND HANDLING... **53**

WHY THE HOLISTIC AND COMPLIANCE APPROACH?.. 53
PRINCIPLES OF HOLISTIC CARE 55
Code of Conduct.. 56
Recognising values.. 58
Respect and dignity in equality & diversity at work 58
COMPONENTS OF HOLISTIC CARE.. 59
Self-care 59
Communication.. 60
Confidentiality... 61
Reporting 62
Safeguarding.. 63
Fluids and nutrition 64
Infections.. 65
Compliance with COSHH 2002 66
Emergency procedures in the workplace 67
CARING IN A HOLISTIC WAY.. 70

Moving & Handling of People in Care Settings

CHAPTER FOUR 71

HUMAN BACK, INJURIES AND DISEASES 71

    THE BIOMECHANICS OF HUMAN MOVEMENT AND THE BACK 71
        Biomechanics 71
        Purpose of the back... 72
        Human torso 72
        Vertebral column 73
        Structure of the back/components 74
        Damage to the spine 76
    MSDS 77
        The symptoms of MSDs.. 78
        Back pain... 78
        Spinal cord injury... 78
        Emergency procedure in back/neck injury 80
        Other Injuries and accidents in the workplace and types 80
    ILLNESSES AND DISABILITY IMPACTING MOVING AND HANDLING............................ 81
        Physical illnesses 81
        Mental illnesses.. 82
        Children and young persons 83
        Learning disability 84
        Some statistics and costs of injuries.. 85

CHAPTER FIVE 87

MANUAL HANDLING OF OBJECTS... 87

    OBJECTS HANDLING ACTIVITIES AND PRINCIPLES 87
        Manual handling activities.. 87
        Manual handling guidelines.. 88
        Principles and techniques of manual handling of inanimate objects..... 89
        Other types of manual lift 91
        Other safety guidelines 93
    TYPES OF RISK ASSESSMENT IN MOVING AND HANDLING 94
        A. Manual Handling Assessment Charts (MAC) tool 94
        B. Risk Assessment of Pushing and Pulling (RAPP) tool 95
        C. Full risk assessment... 96
        Risks and controls in manual handling (objects and people) 96

Moving & Handling of People in Care Settings

Factors influencing risk reduction 100

CHAPTER SIX 101

MOVING AND HANDLING OF PEOPLE 101

MOVING AND HANDLING OF PEOPLE'S ACTIVITIES 101
The principles of moving and handling people 102
Strategy for moving and handling people 103
Common moving and handling situations 103
Special moving and handling situations 107
Personal care 111
UNSAFE / CONTROVERSIAL LIFTING TECHNIQUES 112
Other lifting safety guidelines 118
SUPPORT & COMFORT AIDS 118
List 119
Selected aids/equipment and safe practices 120
HOISTING 127
Hoisting legislation 127
Hoisting risk assessment 128
Hoisting Environment 129
Hoisting checklist and additional guidance according to Legislation . 129
Hoisting guidelines 132

CHAPTER SEVEN 137

TRAINING & PROFESSIONAL DEVELOPMENT 137

KNOWLEDGE, UNDERSTANDING AND SKILLS IN MANUAL HANDLING OF OBJECTS 137
Importance of skills acquisition in manual handling 137
Research 138
The organisational management 139
The Trainer 140
Mandatory Training 141
LEGISLATION AND STRATEGIES FOR TRAINING IN MOVING AND HANDLING 142
Legislation on manual handling training 142
Suggested Holistic Lesson Plan 143
Training tips 144
Examples of practical demonstration and assessment 145
OTHER MATTERS FOR CONSIDERATION 146

Moving & Handling of People in Care Settings

> *Recommended further training after induction* 146
> *Factors that may impact moving and handling in the future* 146
> EMPLOYING ORGANISATION 146
> TRAINING RECORDS 147
>> *Individual learning record* 147
>> *Training Agreement* 147
>> *Workbook* 148
>> *Training certificate* 148

CHAPTER EIGHT 149

CONCLUSION 149

> IN SUMMARY 149
> BIBLIOGRAPHY 152
> ORGANISATIONS THAT SUPPORT BETTER MOVING AND HANDLING OF PEOPLE 155
> INDEXES 157

7 | *Holistic Training Guide*

Moving & Handling of People in Care Settings

Acronyms & Abbreviations

ACOP	Approved Code of Practice
BMA	British Medical Association
Care Certificate	An agreed set of standards defining the knowledge, skills and behaviours expected of CQC-specific job roles in the health and social care sector
CA2014	The Care Act of 2014
CIPD	Chartered Institute of Personnel and Development
COSHH	Control of Substances Hazardous to Health Regulations 2002
CPD	Continuing Professional Development
CQC	Care Quality Commission
CSA2002	Care Standards Act 2002
CSTF	Skills for Health Core Skills Training Framework
DPA	Data Protection Act
DoLS	Deprivation of Liberty Safeguards
GDPR	General Data Protection Regulations 2018
HIW	Healthcare Inspectorate (Wales)
HSE	Health and Safety Executive
HSWA	Health and Safety at Work etc Act 1974
ICO	Information Commissioner's Office
LOLER	Lifting Operations and Lifting Equipment Regulations 1998
LPS	Liberty Protection Safeguards
MAC	Manual Handling Assessment Charts
MHOR	Manual Handling Operations Regulations 1992
MHRA	Medicines and Health Regulatory Authority
MHSWR	Management of Health and Safety at Work Regulations 1999
MSDs	Musculoskeletal disorders
NBE	National Back Exchange
NHS	National Health Service
OFSTED	Office for Standards in Education
ONS	The Office of National Statistics
OSR	The Office for Statistics Regulations
PDP	Personal Development Plan

Moving & Handling of People in Care Settings

PPE	Personal Protective Equipment
PUWER	The Provision and Use of Work Equipment Regulations 1998
RAPP	Risk Assessment of Pushing and Pulling
RIDDOR	Reporting of Injuries, Diseases and Dangerous Occurrences Regulations 2013
RCN	Royal College of Nursing
SWL	Safe Working Load

Moving & Handling of People in Care Settings

Glossary of Terms

Agreed Ways of Working are the policies, procedures, and codes of conduct the organisation provides its workers.
Care and Support enable people to do basic daily life tasks such as getting out of bed, dressing, going to work, cooking meals, seeing friends, caring for their families, and being part of the communities. It can mean emotional support during difficulty, stress, or support from community groups or networks.
Collaboration is about working with someone to achieve a common goal.
Continuing Professional Development is a way of continuing to learn and develop throughout a career, keeping knowledge and skills up to date and safe and effective working.
Competence comprises knowledge, skills, abilities, and attitudes to practise safely and effectively without direct supervision.
Consent is the voluntary acceptance of an appropriately informed person who can agree to the intervention on their behalf.
Dignity includes aspects of daily life such as respect, privacy, autonomy and self-worth. It is also about interpersonal behaviours as well as systems and processes.
Discrimination can result from prejudice, misconception, stereotyping, or a negative attitude. The service user should not be discriminated against based on their protected characteristics, identified explicitly in the Equality Act of 2010. These are race, religion, sex, sexual orientation, age, disability, gender reassignment, marriage/civil partnership or pregnancy/maternity.
Diversity is appreciating and respecting the visible and non-visible differences and values in everyone.
Effective is a success in producing a desired or intended result.
Equality is about equality in opportunities, status, and rights. It does not necessarily mean sameness.
Guide/manual are used interchangeably. Much of the recommendations in the training section of this book can be regarded as a guide, and the entire book is a manual.
Inclusion ensures that people are treated equally, fairly, and inclusively.

Moving & Handling of People in Care Settings

Needs are conditions requiring supply or relief for physical, social, emotional, mental health, and spiritual purposes manifesting in terms of care support.

Personal Development Plan records information on agreed knowledge, skills and behaviour objectives for development, and proposed activities to meet those objectives.

Respect is to have due regard for someone's feelings, wishes or rights.

Reporting is an agreed way of working expressed through a verbal or written account that records adverse events, incidents, errors and issues.

Safe Working Load is the maximum load a lifting equipment can safely carry without fear of breaking down or causing an injury.

Self-care is what people do for themselves and their families to have physical, mental, and general well-being. This refers to practices undertaken by people to manage their own care needs.

Significant Others are colleagues and other professionals across health and social care. *See Chapter One for more details.*

Well-being or a person's well-being includes their sense of hope, confidence, self-esteem, ability to communicate wants and needs or show warmth and affection, experience and pleasure or enjoyment.

Whistleblowing: when a worker reports suspected wrongdoing at work. Officially, this is called 'disclosing the public interest' and may sometimes be called 'escalating concerns.' Workers must report things they feel are not right or illegal or if anyone at work neglects their duties.

Worker is sometimes used interchangeably for a care worker.

Adapted from Skills for Care and Skills for Health

Acknowledgement

Claritas Publishing and Books® is a strategic writing establishment in education, people development, and entertainment. Its contributors also play consulting and management roles in regulated sectors such as health and safety, education and mental health in the workplace. Amongst their professional memberships include the NBE and CIPD.

Copyright & Trademark:
This guide is part of a publication series protected under the registered trademarks of Claritas Publishing and Books® and UK copyright laws. It culminates in years of diverse field experience, training, coaching, and health and social care research.

Credits:
This guide 'contains public sector information published by the Health and Safety Executive and licensed under the Open Government Licence'.[1]

Illustrations in this manual come from Ryan Artwork (pp. 105, 106, 109-111, 113-118 & 128) and Claritas Publishing Limited library (pp. 14, 29, 30, 53, 72, 73, 88, 102, 134-137 & 149) and others from open sources.

Appreciation:
In a further acknowledgement to those who provided expert, structural support and encouragement to make this endeavour a reality, thanks to Rebecca Efeotor for a foreword and a personnel development opportunity to the author to consult and train at Supreme Care Services Ltd over many years. Dr Stephen Ovuefe read and corrected the manuscript, whilst Katarina and George provided the essential moral support to complete this work. Many thanks also go to those the author has met professionally in the moving and handling sector, care service management, and statutory bodies.

A.A. Jude

---

[1] https://www.nationalarchives.gov.uk/doc/open-government-licence/version/3/

Moving & Handling of People in Care Settings

Foreword

Those working in the UK's health and social care industry and those of us with oversight or responsibilities for its management are primarily passionate about what we do. As a regulated activity, we cannot afford to be complacent with moving and handling.

It is, however, not enough to be passionate. It is also about doing what is right. To do what is right, we all must be guided, and the guiding instruments are resources on legislation and directives, policies and procedures that we as service providers set up as agreed ways of working to make everyone in the workplace safe. These policies and procedures must be user-friendly for workers, staff and management in the industry.

This is why this manual is handy and has been published at the appropriate time when coming out of the COVID-19 pandemic; we all need a fresh view and reminder for best practices.

I have read and used many manuals and instructions to develop our staff at Supreme Care Services. What I find different in *Moving and Handling of People in Care Settings: A Holistic and Compliance Manual Handling Training Guide* is its simple tone and holistic approach, applying various aspects of care to the challenges of mobility that care workers and care service users face in combined efforts to attain physical well-being.

This manual will change workers' attitudes rather than only teach them the mechanics of aid and equipment.

This book has been compiled to a high standard by a highly respected trainer with a deep knowledge of manual handling. I recommend this book to those passionate about care who wish to promote doing right for those with physical needs.

Rebecca Efeotor, *Managing Director, Supreme Care Services Ltd., UK*

Chapter One
Introduction

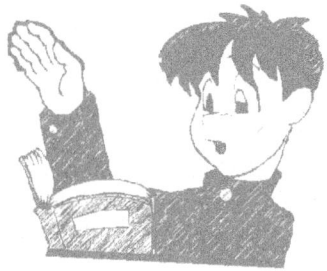

About this Manual

Compliance with the law as a dilemma and solution
During a health and social care training session, this author asked the class about legislation and compliance: "How do you know when you are doing what is right? Is it when you follow the law, your service user is happy, or your employer commends you for your work?" One brain-teasing answer was, "You only have to know the law but always do what is right, depending on whom you are dealing with!" After some discussions around the subject, a dilemma was apparent for the workers. However, this right/proper and legality question arises in the health and care sector and other regulated industries.

The added complexion of this puzzle in moving and handling people is that a handling worker not only has a legal obligation to the individuals but also must follow specific organisations' procedures and manufacturers' guidelines for moving aids and equipment they operate. It seems a "triple-whammy" compliance dilemma.

Many, however, often ignore that the law protects the worker

Moving & Handling of People in Care Settings

more than it is credited. The support from organisations, service users, and their families could sometimes be shifty.

For the law, it is often a case of zero-tolerance for wrongdoing, and rightly so, particularly on safeguarding matters. For care organisations, without which the entire health and social care system may collapse, there are unending financial pressures to employ, retain and develop good care workers. For the service users and their families, it is a case of value for their money, either paid by the state or not.

For care workers, however, most people are oblivious to their rights to work in a suitable and safe environment. This is particularly so for those responsible for moving and handling people. It is within the context of this suitable and safe environment that this book has meaning as a compliance manual.

Moving and handling people is regulated because it is core to the health and social care sector and because specific legal codes cover it as an activity.

This manual follows the "approved Code of Practice (ACOP) and associated guidance" on complying with the following health and safety legislation:
1. the *Lifting Operations and Lifting Equipment Regulations 1998*" (LOLER Regulation 5);
2. the relevant moving and handling activities provisioned in the *Health and Safety at Work etc Act 1974* (HSWA Regulation 3);
3. the Provision and Use of Work Equipment Regulations 1998 (PUWER Regulations 4, 8, 9); and

4. the *Management of Health and Safety at Work Regulations 1999* (MHSWR Regulation 19).
All as set out by the HSE.

The HSE has the authority to set out the ACOP with the consent of the parliament through the Secretary of State. With its legal status, one can be prosecuted for a breach under the health and safety laws. It is on this authority and this authority only that this guide essentially relies upon.

Existing manuals, handbooks and guides
There are very good manuals and guides on general or specific subjects in manual handling, a few of which this author has reviewed. Some resources provide frameworks for reputable organisations, whilst several are approved and used by well-known occupational practitioners and skills training service providers for health and social care workers. Notable examples are guidelines used by the NBE and the RCN.[2]

Unlike most of these resources, however, this manual provides handy, easy-to-assimilate support for care workers, carers, employers, and organisations facing legal compliance challenges. If collaboration is critical in the health and social care sector, a resource should also allow stakeholders to know the fundamental (legal) challenges facing other stakeholders with whom they should collaborate: a broad appeal of this manual.

Another focus of this book not found in pre-pandemic resources is the consideration of the impact of COVID-19 on the care sector; the BMA, in a 2023 Report, confirmed that more

---

[2] https://www.rcn.org.uk/get-help/rcn-advice/moving-and-handling

individuals in care settings and their workers suffered the impact of COVID than the general population.[3] This situation called for a review of the risk of infection in the moving and handling environment.

A more significant difference between *Moving and Handling of People in Care Settings: A Holistic and Compliance Manual Handling Training Guide* and other resources is that this adopts a **holistic** approach to moving and handling, putting in clear context components of **well-being** as set out in the Care Act of 2014 (CA2014) and meeting with the requirements of all essential core and bye-laws of Health and Safety at Work etc Act 1974 (HSWA) to make everyone safe in the workplace.

The reader will enjoy a subtle presentation of the importance of meeting service users' "varied" needs, such as safeguarding, consent, communication, diversity, fluids nutrition and infection control, which are indeed consequential to their moving and handling from the perspective of workers' duty of care.

Finally, it is pertinent to note that the term 'moving and handling' is sometimes commonly used in the health sector, while 'moving and positioning' is sometimes used in social care. No distinction is made between these two terms in this manual.

Who should read this manual?
Moving and Handling of People in Care Settings: A Holistic and Compliance Manual Handling Training Guide is helpful for care workers and stakeholders who support them in moving and handling service users, particularly those with a duty of care.

---

[3] BMA, 2023 Report, *The impact of the pandemic on population health and health inequalities,* London. pp15-17.

In achieving this:
1. It recognises the difference between care workers and generally unpaid carers.
2. It recognises organisations as employers and specifies, where possible, mid and senior-level staff, such as supervisors and health and safety managers who send workers and health professionals into the fields or manage their care homes or health facilities.
3. It will guide those responsible for policy and procedure reviews within organisations.
4. In addition, it is helpful for duty-holders with responsibilities for moving and handling aids and equipment, local authority personnel or occupational professionals who may collaborate with workers in the workplace to bring about best practices in moving and handling, and well-being.

This manual does not pretend to cover all aspects of moving and handling; however, it can support organisations in setting up supervision plans and streamlining policies and procedures.

It will also assist in planning, developing, and reviewing their training to avoid safeguarding issues and cope with service users' mobility challenges.

In conclusion, this manual is helpful for those who train at induction, refresher, or intervention levels in the health and social care sector to impart knowledge and improve workers' handling of individuals with varied challenges.

<u>The Manual's objectives</u>
A reader should:

1. Understand legislation in moving and handling people for compliance.
2. Understand employers' and employees' responsibilities and legal duties.
3. Promote holistic care and support.
4. Understand unsafe manual handling risk factors, including posturing and how injuries can occur.
5. Promote back care.
6. Understand relevant basic risk assessment approaches.
7. Increase standards around single-handed care.
8. Support training for all the above.
9. Understand the dynamics of stakeholders' collaboration.
10. Support policy and procedure process in moving and handling.

The structure

Chapter One continues with the definitions and meanings of some standard terms to avoid differing interpretations by readers. It concludes by identifying the care sector stakeholders responsible for best practices and those with legal obligations. It underscores the importance of collaboration for the well-being of service users.

Chapter Two sets out an understanding of moving and handling within the general context of manual handling and the associated consequences of poor handling. It discusses relevant legislation and issues in care settings to avoid legal pitfalls.

Chapter Three is dedicated to understanding the holistic approach in care and how it impacts the moving and handling of people, setting out the components of this approach and their applications.

Moving & Handling of People in Care Settings

In Chapter Four, the manual discusses the importance of the human back, its biomechanics, MSDs, injuries and accidents in the workplace as they impact care workers and their service users.

Chapter Five is dedicated to manually handling inanimate objects, discussing the common principles of moving and handling from perspectives of knowledge, understanding, skills and safety guidelines on practical matters. A broad overview of risk assessment and risk control guidelines follows later and concludes this chapter.

In contrast, Chapter Six focuses on the moving and handling of people and its principles, strategy, and techniques. It identifies some controversial handling techniques whilst listing the activity's common aids and equipment and discusses the usage and safety guidelines for a few aids, particularly the hoist.

The penultimate chapter, Seven, is dedicated to training, providing information to support trainers in planning and delivering knowledge and skills and promoting behaviours pertinent to a safe, person-centred-focused workplace. A summary follows this in the final chapter.

Selected Terms Definitions

Employee
A person retained for wages or salary to undertake care service on behalf of an employer. They participate in moving and handling activities in the workplace by being physically present in the service user's home or remotely from the employer's workplace.

Some legislation in Chapter Two sets out the obligations of employees, and their role as stakeholders is often linked to their employers' responsibilities.

Employer
A legal entity, person, or firm, also known as the organisation that retains people for care service. An employer has control over lifting equipment to a defined extent. Its employees include supervisors or care service managers. This definition also applies where there may not be a direct 'employment' relationship between the service user and the person who controls the lifting equipment. An example is an equipment hire company using the organisation's workplace or another person's premises on behalf of the organisation.

Employers' requirements imposed by moving and handling regulations also apply to self-employed people. Organisations still have responsibilities that involve using third parties or even other self-employed people for their services.

This definition does not apply to those selling or leasing lifting equipment. Some legislations in Chapter Two set out the obligations of employers.

Lifting equipment[4]
According to HSE, lifting equipment is "work equipment for lifting or lowering loads and includes anchoring, fixing or supporting attachments". In the case of an example like a **hoist** that is used for lifting, lowering and placing service users, this definition includes accessories such as the **hoist battery**; other aids that "attach a load", such as the **sling**; an "aid used to

---

[4] LOLER. https://www.hse.gov.uk/work-equipment-machinery/loler.htm

support" the hoist in the lifting such as a **sliding sheet,** or the **railing track** in the case of an overhead hoist.

Lifting operation
A lifting operation is an operation concerned with the lifting or lowering of a load. LOLER Regulation 8 (2).

Load
A 'load' is the item or items being lifted, which includes a person or people.[5] LOLER Regulation 8 (2).

Manual handling operations
According to MHOR, "manual handling operations" means transporting or supporting a load (including lifting, putting down, pushing, pulling, carrying or moving) by hand or bodily force.[6]

An Overview of Stakeholders in Moving and Handling

The individual or service user
Service users are those directly affected by the services provided by a regulated care service provider. Also known as individuals, service users may be commonly called patients in health care settings. A service user is not necessarily a client, particularly those under the care of the state, though this term is often used to describe them. Service users are generally deemed vulnerable by law.

More and more people are being cared for at home due to

---

[5] https://books.hse.gov.uk/LOLER
[6] https://lead-academy.org/blog/illegal-moving-and-handling-techniques/

Moving & Handling of People in Care Settings

dependency needs, dignity awareness, and quicker hospital discharges resulting from better health treatments that make people live longer. Lack of funding can also cause hospital decongestions.

According to Age UK, 1.5m older people need care. *NHS Digital, 2022, Adult Social Care Statistics in England: An Overview* adds further care requests of 1.3m for those above 65 and 611,000 for those between 18 and 64 years. Care needs may vary depending on the age or severity of the illness, and these needs may be short, medium, or long-term.

Service users cut across socio-cultural divides, but young people's care requires additional training and vetting.

The carer and the care worker
A carer who looks after an ill, disabled, or older person at home is not bound by a care worker's legal obligations (duty of care). They are, however, by general harm-prevention laws.

According to *Carers UK* (2022), there are 10.6m carers in the UK, most of whom face enormous challenges in supporting individuals with mobility issues compared to care workers. Eighty per cent are females, 27% have a disability themselves, and the majority are aged between 45 and 54 years. While carers are primarily unpaid, only 41% are employed, though the government may recognise their roles and provide them with some social or financial benefits. Most carers are relatives or acquaintances of an individual needing care, but a volunteer carer may be engaged to look after a person if there is no friend or relative to act as a carer.

A volunteer carer can also support a home carer who may need

Moving & Handling of People in Care Settings

to take time off or provide tasks that a home carer cannot carry out alone, as in double-handed care in the paid care sector. People of all ages can volunteer to become carers.

Carers collaborate with care workers concerning moving and handling. However, unlike their paid counterparts, they do not routinely receive formal training on moving and handling other than informal sessions that occupational therapists sometimes provide to guide the correct operation of moving and handling equipment.

Care workers have obligations to look after their health; however, it is worth noting that according to statistics, about 66% of carers report that they are in fair or bad physical health, while up to 75% report fair or bad mental health.[7]

Furthermore, care workers are persons employed with the legal duty to support a service user. In other words, they are duty-holders who help service users retain as much independence as possible. Apart from the professional conduct expected of them, care work is a difficult task that requires skill and sensitivity, for which they must be trained. According to *The ONS 2020*, there are 3.06m care workers in the UK.[8]

By the end of 2019, the adult care sector was experiencing significant staffing pressures. Workforce shortages were around "122,000, with 1,100 people estimated to leave their job daily – an annual leaver rate of almost a third – and a quarter of staff

---

[7] Carers UK, *State of Caring 2022: A snapshot of unpaid care in the UK*, November 2022. p.34.
[8] Office for National Statistics (ons.gov.uk)

on a zero-hours contract".[9]

Care workers' duty, roles, obligations and responsibilities are defined in the Care Certificate Standards.[10] Below is a summary.

Duty of a care worker
Duty is the legal obligation to all at the workplace. It has two goals:
1. Promote well-being.
2. Protect from abuse, neglect, harm or exploitation.

Role of a care worker
1. Provide care to improve service users' well-being.
2. Support service users' wishes for independence.
3. Work to respect service users' values.
4. Keep service users physically comfortable.
5. Collaborate with other care workers and Significant Others.
6. Be a worthy ambassador for their organisation, contributing to activities.
7. Avoid using their attitudes and values to override service users' needs.
8. Respect the confidentiality of the records and other information of services.

(It should be observed that these roles are workers' direct obligations to service users.)

Other Obligations and responsibilities of a care worker
1. Maintain physical and mental well-being by eating a

---

[9] Ben Gershlick, B and Charlesworth, A., 2019, "Health and social care workforce: Priorities for the next government". The Health Foundation.
[10] Care Certificate (skillsforcare.org.uk).

proper diet, resting well, exercising and learning to deal with stress.
2. Follow the procedure and do not work outside the care or handling plan.
3. Follow professional and approved codes of practice.
4. Follow the organisation's policy and procedure, including whistleblowing.
5. Follow safeguarding rules.
6. Promote self-development and develop professionally through training and qualifications.
7. Be prepared for emergencies.
8. Keep accurate records of work activities.
9. Always work with a person-centred approach.

The employer/organisation
Obligations to the service user
1. Subscribe to the HSE ACOP to ensure the highest possible standards of care and protect the rights and welfare of the service users.
2. Comply with regulations of service users' safety and well-being.

Obligations to employees
1. Keep their side of the agreement made with employees.
2. Provide adequate training.
3. Be well-guided on workers' rights, including those on zero-hours contracts. The *EC Health and Safety Framework* outlines protection requirements and workers' entitlement to an industrial tribunal "if any action is taken against them by their employer if they leave the workplace because of dangerous

Moving & Handling of People in Care Settings

circumstances or take appropriate steps to protect themselves, or others, from the danger".[11]
4. Encourage workers to keep clear records of adherence to care and handling plans.
5. Have periodic consultations with employees on health and safety matters in the workplace as set out
6. by the HSE.[12]
7. Under HSWA provisions, if workers are employed on the basis that they are responsible for their health and safety (self-employed or bank staff, for instance), legal advice should be sought before doing so.

Obligations on new care aids and equipment

Procurement of new aids and equipment for general care or moving and handling, particularly by employers, is encouraged in law but not compulsory.

Regulations require equipment compliance with *Article 100a Product Safety Directive*. Whilst most new lifting equipment will meet this directive, the minimum requirement is usually below the directive, depending on the degree of risk. This is why risk must be assessed in each case. Where there are risks of contamination or infections, new aids must be procured.

Other compliance requirements
1. Legislation, including confidentiality, safeguarding, statutory, etc.
2. Adequate business insurance to cover liabilities.

---

[11] The European Framework Directive on Safety and Health at Work (Directive 89/391 EEC) adopted in 1989.
[12] HSE, 2013, *Consulting employees on health and safety: A brief guide to the law*, INDG232 (rev2).

Trainers

Moving and handling regulations make workers' training mandatory, and it is an offence for an organisation not to provide its staff with training that will be commensurate with their assigned tasks.

Trainers are highly recommended not to be involved with the care organisation's day-to-day administration or management; however, there could be visits to service users to assess workers' performances or adherence to the organisation's policies and procedures.

To visit service users, trainers must be DBS-checked and without conflict of interest.

Training could be in-house and outsourced. In either case, trainers should adapt resources to suit the organisation's policies and procedures, separating induction, refresher and corrective or intervention sessions. The latter is necessary when statutory or regulatory agencies identify shortcomings or needs for an organisation to correct or improve care.

Organisations should train workers, supervisors, and managers in moving and handling to know what updates are in the industry.

Significant Others

A worker or their organisation may be required to collaborate with other professionals who have responsibilities or obligations to the service user or to improve care service. Such collaborators are referred to as Significant Others and may consist of:

> **Social workers** are responsible for the needs of the

service users, carers, and care workers. They compile and award the packages and monitor the care service provided. They may inform statutory authorities if things go wrong. They also have specific legal obligations to initiate or respond to policies to ensure safety within the care environment.

Healthcare professionals such as GPs and nurses who provide general medical advice, treatment, and support. They may physically intervene by attending the home or asking for the service user to be brought to surgery or the hospital for health care.

Mental health professionals such as mental health nurses or psychiatrists support the service users and others with mental disorders or disabilities through counselling, support or writing reports.

Occupational therapists who assess the service user's aids and equipment requirements and how their homes can be adapted for equipment and activities to enable them to relearn skills for independence.

Physiotherapists that treat those with bone and joint problems while advising on mobility and exercise.

Statutory Organisations could be social, health or governmental agencies such as the CQC, local authorities, or the OFSTED. They are legally responsible for assessing care services and licensing or providing legal or statutory guidance or policies for compliance. They also investigate and punish wrongdoings or failures.

Chapter Two
The Legislation

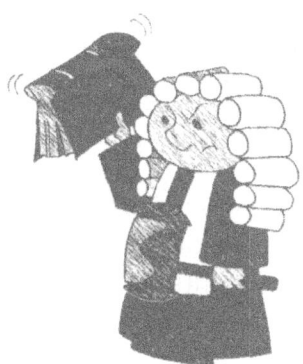

Understanding Manual Handling and Moving and Handling of People

Manual handling and moving and handling
According to MHOR, manual handling applies to activities involving the transporting or supporting loads, including lifting, lowering, pushing, pulling, carrying or moving loads where loads are inanimate, for example, a box or a trolley, or animate, for example, a person.

The same law singles out "moving and handling" as a specific manual handling activity that deals with people.

In previous years, it was all about manual handling when it was erroneously accepted that people could be 'manually handled'. With the technology surrounding moving equipment not as advanced as it is now, it was not difficult to see where the problems laid. There were what would now be deemed unsafe manual handling practices, particularly in handling people.

There obviously needed to be a difference between moving loads such as boxes and moving people. There are no better ways to understand the similarities and differences between manual handling and moving and handling than the bases provided in legislation and risk assessment.

On similarities, the legislation focuses on preventing MSDs and promoting risk assessments that create a safe environment and activity. On differences, MHOR clarifies the issues in the context of the worker, their environment, the load and the risk they face. Concerning handling people, the law focuses on the risk to the care worker and their service users.

Risk assessments for both inanimate objects and people differ from the perspective that manual handling of objects follows a general assessment of the environmental setting, whilst moving and handling risk assessment is more people-focused.

It is now more acceptable to refer to the relevant people-focused activity as moving and handling rather than manual handling, particularly when some activities related to handling people have either been deemed unsafe or controversial for further use. Some of these unsafe techniques are discussed in Chapter Six.

The general purposes of relevant legislation
Manual handling legislation is enacted chiefly to prevent harm and promote safety. It is, therefore, firm on the need for risk assessment to achieve these purposes, particularly when some moving and handling activities may involve incorrect but avoidable posturing, such as bending, twisting, and static drooping positions and decisions. Outcomes of the use of non-compliant equipment may also not be as anticipated. Risk

assessment is a way of managing activities with uncertain outcomes.

For a care worker, wrong decisions and uncertain outcomes from non-compliant equipment may fall foul of the law. This lack of compliance can impact the worker and their colleagues' financial, physical, and mental well-being and, of course, the service user, with devastating consequences ranging from loss of life to loss of income and disruption to family life. While the duty for a safe workplace is mostly the employer's, care workers are responsible for keeping themselves and others safe. The decision to work in safety is ultimately theirs to make.

Legislation in Moving and Handling

MHOR 1992 / 2002
Manual Handling Operations Regulation is a 1992 regulation that enforces a European Manual Handling Directive (amended in 2002), supporting the HSWA. It regulates requirements to be made concerning manual handling with concerns for the risks of injury from manual handling operations. The law aims to reduce the "incidence and prevalence of MSDs arising from the manual handling of loads at work", and unlike MHSWR, It does not place a duty on carers or volunteer carers.

MHOR Regulation 4 makes clear the employer's duty to:
1. Avoid requiring its employees to undertake any manual handling operations at work that involve a risk of injury.
2. Moreover, if (1) *above* is impossible, make a suitable and sufficient assessment of all such

Moving & Handling of People in Care Settings

    operations.[13]
3. Take appropriate steps to reduce the risk of injury during those operations to the lowest level reasonably practicable.[14]
4. Use a designed assessment strategy to provide at-risk employees with general indications and precise information on the load.

Regulation 4 further seeks to avoid manual handling by eliminating it or using automation or mechanisation.

MHOR Regulation 5 makes clear the employee's duty that:
1. Each working employee should make full and proper use of any system of work provided, and
2. As required by Section 7 of the HSWA, employees must:
  i. Take reasonable care of their health and safety and that of others who may be affected by their activities;
  ii. Co-operate with the employer to comply with their health and safety duties.

MHOR further recognises that workers are at risk if they are:
1. Physically unsuited to carry out the tasks in question.
2. Wearing unsuitable clothing, footwear, or other personal effects.[15]
3. Not having adequate or appropriate knowledge

---

[13] https://www.hse.gov.uk/foi/internalops/ocs/300-399/313_5.htm
[14] The Manual Handling Operations Regulations 1992 (as amended) (MHOR)
[15] *Ibid.*

or training.
3. Not risk-assessing activities or keeping to reviewed changes in assessments.

LOLER 1998

LOLER Regulation 2 places a duty on people and organisations that own, operate, or have control over lifting equipment, as well as employees using such equipment, whether owned by them or not. It also applies to organisations providing lifting equipment for others to control risks and avoid any injury or damage to health and well-being. Organisations must ensure that their contractors comply with this law.

Regulation 4 requires organisations to use the stress test to ensure that lifting equipment is of adequate strength and stability for each load. This is supported by ensuring employers and employees follow the manufacturer's instructions.

Equipment maintenance should be done by competent persons (Regulation 9) who should mark the equipment with labels or stamps (Regulation 7).

For any planned activity, LOLER Regulation 8(1) clarifies that each lifting operation needs to be:
1. properly planned by a competent person;
2. appropriately supervised and
3. carried out safely.

Regulation 9(3)a) requires that equipment used for lifting is not only appropriate or suitable for the task, but it must also fit the purpose, complying with the statutory periodic (6 months) 'thorough examination'. Furthermore, records of all thorough examinations must be kept, and any defects found must be reported to the person responsible for the equipment.

There are some areas that LOLER does not cover, however. They are:
1. The definition of lifting equipment.
    (It ascribes this to PUWER).
2. Potential risks of lifting equipment.
    (It defers this to the safeguards provided in other legislations. For example, the requirement for risk assessment is identified in MHSWR).
3. The acquisition of lifting equipment by members of the public for use in their homes.
4. Where equipment is loaned by a healthcare or community equipment provider for use by the individual or their family, to use such equipment.

(However, the organisation has a duty to ensure the employee's safety).

PUWER 1998

This Regulation seeks to ensure the safety of people and organisations operating, maintaining, and controlling the equipment used in their workplaces. Staff must be trained for the equipment they are assigned to operate.

PUWER places a duty on equipment owners, operators, or those controlling work equipment just as it does on organisations whose employees use such equipment, whether owned by them or not.

The legislation requires that work equipment suits the work to be done to reduce risks to health and safety. Furthermore, equipment should be suitable, safe, maintained and inspected to ensure that it is correctly installed and does not subsequently deteriorate.

To manage health and safety, PUWER defers to the HSWA. Like the 1974 Act, however, Regulation 4(1&2) deals with the safety of work equipment from three aspects: [16]
1. its initial integrity;
2. the place where it will be used and
3. the purpose for which it will be used.

MHSWR 1999
Regulation 3 of this law places a duty on employers and employees to require a risk assessment for their workplace activities involving lifting operations, management of potential risks, and proportionate actions to mitigate identified risks. Risk assessment is a duty. It is a criminal offence for an employer not to 'make a suitable and sufficient assessment'.

The employer must protect employees and others from harm with the following minimum set of actions:
1. Identify what hazards could cause injury or illness in the workplace.
2. Decide how likely someone could be harmed and how seriously (the risk).
3. If this is impossible, take action to eliminate the hazard or control the risk.

MHSWR Regulation 4 requires employers to make a suitable and sufficient assessment of unavoidable hazardous activities, requiring risk assessment staff to be competent, have good operation knowledge, and comply with RIDDOR. The Regulation also commits organisations to this duty based on size, from

---

[16] https://www.hse.gov.uk/foi/internalops/ocs/600-699/oc634_7.htm

small, low-risk organisations to medium and high-risk. It highlights the importance of aids and equipment and their assessments, relevance and safety of use, acknowledging the types of injuries they can cause and, setting the regulations for their maintenance, touching on the necessity of training that focuses on skills, knowledge and experience.

Concerning young people, MHSWR Regulation 19 requires special risk assessment "considerations" for young people even though a special risk assessment template is needed.

HSWA 1974
This Regulation is the UK's primary legislation covering occupational health, welfare, and safety. It sets out the duties of employers and self-employed towards their employees and members of the public.

The employer's duties under HSWA are:
1. Provision and maintenance of aids, equipment, plant, and work systems, avoiding risks.
2. Policies and procedures should be made available for all aspects of work, including manual handling, hazards, accidents, and incidents.
3. Provide necessary information, training, and supervision, ensuring employees' health and safety as reasonably practicable.

The employee's duties under HSWA are:
1. Make themselves, colleagues and others safe.
2. Work safely.
3. Use equipment safely.
4. Exercise the right to refuse a task if there is no "safe system of work".

5. Be willing to receive training.

A duty under the HSWA cannot be passed to others using a contract, and there will still be a duty towards others under Section 3 of the HSWA. An organisation will still be legally responsible where third parties, self-employed, or contractors are employed to undertake activities covered under the HSWA.

RIDDOR 2013
This Regulation requires employers and those in control of work premises to report and keep records of the following:
1. Work-related deaths.
2. Serious injuries.
3. Certain dangerous occurrences (near-miss incidents).

Employers should have a RIDDOR Policy, and employees should be trained on the differences between accidents and incidents. The legal guideline for reporting under health and safety laws is RIDDOR.

Reporting under RIDDOR
1. All accidents or incidents that may occur during a working day must be reported to the Care Manager, no matter how trivial they may seem.
2. The details must be entered into the accident report book in the office.
3. The employer must follow up on the report and identify health and safety issues.
4. Employees must maintain their safety and that of their service users and colleagues.
5. Employees must be vigilant, apply all safety regulations, and act upon the training given.

6. Only 'responsible persons', including employers, should submit reports under RIDDOR. The responsible person is:
   a. an employee whose employer has designated or, in their absence,
   b. the worker present or the person responsible for the workplace.
7. Regarding non-fatal injuries to workers, what is reported should be a work-related accident that significantly damages the body.
8. In the case of work-related fatalities, the responsible person must follow the reporting procedure when any person dies due to a work-related accident.

Reporting template and record-keeping

The incident report should include:
1. The date and time of the accident or dangerous occurrence.
2. The Individual's
   a. full name;
   b. occupation;
   c. injury;
   d. the place where the accident or the dangerous occurrence happened;
   e. brief description of the circumstances in which the accident or dangerous occurrence happened;
   f. the date that the accident or the dangerous occurrence was first reported to the relevant authority and
   g. the method by which the accident or dangerous occurrence was reported.

Care Act 2014

This reforming law governs how adult social care in England should be provided, putting people and their carers in control of their care and support. The Act increases the obligations of local authorities in care by establishing a single, consistent route to an entitlement to public care and support for all adults. It clarifies the distinction between carers and care workers, providing more support than ever for carers.

Promoting the well-being of individuals and protecting them from harm is at the centre of this legislation. The law further entrenches the importance of stakeholders' collaboration with attention to equality and diversity and the care plan with how it should be used in care, emphasising punishment for not following it.

This legislation gives those over 18 who care for the disabled or ill the right to a carer's assessment. This also considers their physical and mental capacity to collaborate with paid care workers.

Section 42 of the Act gives the local authority power to investigate safeguarding breaches, and Section 90 reaffirms the independence of the CQC in regulatory matters. On the education and training of care workers, Sections 97 and 103 of the Act give the Secretary of State duty for Local Education Training Boards to oversee education and training.

Finally, this law signals a holistic approach to care through the concept of well-being.

Other Legal and Compliance Issues in Moving and Handling

Duty of care as a legal obligation
The duty of those engaged in care (employers, employees, and others) is entrenched in relevant manual handling laws, a breach of which can be punished according to the law.

Fulfilment of duty in moving and handling
In the case of a care worker, the duty of care is fulfilled by:
- Safeguarding individuals
- Treating them fairly with respect and dignity
- Protecting their rights
- Giving them a choice
- Supporting their complaints
- Raising concerns and duty reporting (RIDDOR)
- Following the care and handling plans
- Compliance with agreed ways of working
- Collaborating with others

A moving and handling worker must comply with the legislation, policies and procedures that meet the CQC's Fundamental Standards of Quality and Safety.[17] They should also follow the Code of Conduct for England's Healthcare Support Workers and Adult Social Care Workers.[18]

Care plan (and handling plan)
A care plan is a person-centred document combining legislation, policy, and procedure defining the care of a person. Failure to follow a care plan could unintentionally harm the service user, the harm that may come through a worker's actions or

---

[17] www.cqc.org.uk/file/447
[18] *www.skillsforhealth.org.uk/code-of-conduct*

inactions.

The care plan must always be in the service user's home as it contains the information workers need to fulfil their responsibilities to meet the individual's needs. Such information will include details of emergency services, GPs, and other relevant care persons. Organisations should carefully plan and update or review the care plan to prevent loss of care.

A handling plan may be an additional document that details moving and handling activities but is always a part of the overall plan of care.

Reporting and documentation
Reporting and documentation are essential in moving and handling for continuity, well-being and care integrity. Handling procedure to assist in this activity is integrated into the care plan and should be completed as trained. Another integrated procedure may be the Medication Administration Records (MAR) sheets, which must also be completed as the law requires.

The care/handling plan should not record information that could expose the service user to abuse, neglect, harm or exploitation, and the service users have the right to read or see what is written in the document because it belongs to them. The worker's employer will provide training on informing the care/handling plan.

No pages of the care/handling plan should be unilaterally removed without the agreement of stakeholders; mistakes must be rectified on the same page.

Reporting mistakes

As humans, we make mistakes, and as such, in care, there should be an honest reporting of mistakes such as adverse events, errors, near misses, and workplace incidents according to the organisation's policy so that:
- Corrective actions are taken, and
- Lessons are learnt

Policy and procedure
Organisations must have approved policies and procedures for activities that should be made known at induction. These policies and procedures are derived from legislation or other by-laws and guidelines set out by statutory bodies. They are also supposed to incorporate best practices in the industry.

An organisation needs to have a policy on every aspect of care delivery. Few organisations claim no-lifting policies concerning moving and handling without explaining to workers what that could be or training on what such a procedure would entail. Policies and procedures also need to be reviewed periodically.

Ergonomic risk assessment process in moving and handling
Moving and handling is a regulated activity. Much of the relevant laws outlined in the previous section place duty on employers and employees on risk assessments, generally and particularly in moving and handling, because every activity or workplace has potentially specific accident health hazards and risks.

Further guidance on risk assessments can be found in *Risk assessment: A brief guide to controlling risks in the workplace* INDG163. This document pays attention to accident hazards and risks and improves designs, comfort and performance of aids and equipment. In other words, risk assessments have led to technological advances in the workplace.

Risk assessment and technological advances

Technological advances emanating from ergonomic risk assessment processes are applied to the organisational, cognitive, and physical parameters of aids and equipment. In other words, modern equipment enables workers to be better organised in their responsibilities and manage the equipment with basic or minimum skill requirements. Equipment tends to be sleeker, less bulky, more portable and supposedly effective.

These have resulted in better activity performance, comfort, ease of use, aesthetic designs, safety features, and cost reduction. A good example would be a wheelchair that can double up as a commode or a foldable or mobile hoist with low voltage and better safety features than previous types.

General headings checklist to eliminate or reduce hazards:

Biological	Chemical
Electrical	Environmental
Fire	Handling
Lifting	Mechanical
Physical	Stress
Height and weight	Communication and comprehension
Handling constraints	Assessment of specific skills
Level of assistance needed	Specific equipment needed

Areas of consideration for risk assessment are:

Task	The capability of the individual
Load	Environment
Equipment	Young people
Single or double-handed care	Local authority policy

Basic principles in risk assessment

- Identifying risks
- Evaluating risks
- Deciding who is at risk
- Rating the risk
- Assessing before acting
- Complying with the law
- Ready to provide evidence to the watchdogs such as HSE and statutory organisations such as CQC and Local Authority
- Managing risk assessment to address hazard problems or issues
- Recording assessment
- Reviewing assessment

Other issues to consider in Risk Assessment

- Assessments should be done in the service user's home.

Abuse

Abuse occurs in a relationship of expectation of trust that causes harm or injury to another person, thereby violating their human or civil rights. Abuse can be either intentionally or inadvertently inflicted.

Organisations should be aware of institutional abuse where procedures are not legally compliant or training violates regulations. A worker operating within such an environment may abuse service users advertently or inadvertently.

Abuse has severe safeguarding implications and is punishable by law. As workers carry out their responsibilities in an environment of trust, they should be trained in safeguarding, particularly the different types of abuse, with a particular understanding of physical abuse and the legal use of restraints in handling service users. Their training should also enable them to identify abuses by family members or non-duty-holders attending the workplace.

Four common types of abuse in moving and handling
1. **Physical**: this is cited where the service user is physically harmed, injured, or hurt, for example, hitting the knee on the hoist or aggravated pressure/bed sores through turning falls.

    Bruises sustained through rough, non-delicate handling may be deemed abuse if not reported. Any intention to inflict such harm is punishable by law.

    Workers should pay attention to unexplained bruises on the service users and report them accordingly, and neither should they cover up any such bruises they may cause to the service user.

2. **Neglect**: where there is the presence of the individual's unmet needs, such as food, drink, medication, personal care or on-time transfer to required positions. Neglect is a failure or omission to act or do the right thing. Failure

to move a service user as required by the handling plan is neglect.

Service users likewise cannot self-neglect on their care by refusing needs to harm themselves. Persistent refusal to accept care should be reported. A service user refusing to be moved from one position to a more comfortable, healthier or safer position may be committing self-neglect.

3. **Emotional/psychological**: where the service user, for instance, feeling withdrawn, unloved, unsecured, or inadequate may be signs of emotional or psychological abuse.

   Care workers should look for signs of very distressing moving and handling activities. The individuals must not be distressed before engaging in the activities without the care worker enquiring about the causes or reporting accordingly.

4. **Institutional**: where there are poor care standards, rigid routines, ineffective training, or failure by the organisation and staff to provide the proper care, support and information. Poor working conditions and staff morale affect workers' activity at the workplace, and the service users may be harmed by such. Workers must be involved in reviews of handling activities.

Workers should guard against other types of abuse found in the workplace, such as financial, discriminatory or sexual that may hinder a service user's cooperation during moving and handling activities. Their training should equip them to understand the signs of these abuses and how to deal with them.

Consent

The CQC requires organisations' knowledge and understanding of Regulation 11 of the Health and Social Care Act 2008 (Regulated Activities) Regulations 2014 on training and assessments for moving and handling workers.

Workers and care managers should be trained and reminded that care and treatment of service users must only be provided with the service user's consent. Those lacking the capacity to give such consent should be registered, and workers must act in accordance with the Mental Capacity Act 2005 (MCA) in providing their care.

Workers should realise that every moving and handling activity requires seeking the service user's consent when informing them of the proposed or pending care activity. Workers should provide this information with clarity and conciseness so that the service user understands without ambiguity. Such information should also include the possible risks, complications, and any alternatives to the activity. This is one reason that communication skills are essential for moving and handling care activities.

Consent must be treated as a continuous process throughout a care activity, and workers should beware that consent may be withheld or withdrawn by the individual at any time. If a legally named advocate gives consent on behalf of the service user, all workers must respect this.

Deprived liberties

Consents are linked to Deprivation of Liberty Safeguards (DoLS), soon-to-be Liberty Protection Safeguards (LPS), a least restrictive MCA tool that removes or limits one's liberty in specific situations to meet their needs to protect them from severe harm where there is a lack of capacity to make a safe decision for oneself.

DoLS will mostly apply in hospitals or care homes with the approval of local authorities or in a domiciliary setting with permission of the Court of Protection. Workers should understand that they cannot force any service user into any moving and handling activity without establishing DoLS.

A worker would know if an individual's liberties have been deprived, meaning that other named persons must decide on their basic needs.

The CQC or the HIW monitors DoLS in England and Wales, respectively.

Mental Capacity Act 2005
The MCA provides a better understanding of the capacity to make decisions and establishes that decisions or choices made should be informed. In moving and handling, for instance, informed choice requires that care workers clearly and fully provide all information surrounding the activity, including an explanation of the process, while not omitting the positives and negatives of the process.

MCA posits that all individuals have the right to make their own decisions. However, the regulation establishes that there are situations where individuals can no longer make their own decisions because they have a condition affecting their cognition. MCA further provides a methodology to establish this lack of capacity. Few service users will fall into this category.

This process is based on five principles:
1. Think or accept that the service user can make a decision.
2. Give all practical support to help them make that decision.
3. Do not say they cannot decide because their decision or a previous decision was wrong.
4. When someone is named to decide for them, the decision must be the best of the available options.
5. When someone is named to decide for them, the decision must be the least restrictive of the available options.

Where decisions are made for them, the care/handling plan will state clearly who the Advocate is or set out the decision-making procedure. In moving and handling, MCA principles go to the heart of getting the service user's consent each time during the activity process.

Work ethics
The care/handling worker is invited to follow good work ethics, including:
1. Sensitivity, reliability, equality, diversity and recognition that service users are entitled to have value for their money.
2. Professionalism and always thinking of the needs of service users.
3. Maintaining the service user's dignity, respect, and confidentiality. This particularly manifests in how

workers touch the individuals during the moving and handling process.
4. Working with Significant Others.
5. Honesty in the workplace.
6. Positive response to training.
7. Following the organisation's procedure.

Emergency care and first aid

Emergency care and First Aid are part of a holistic approach to moving and handling. See Chapter Three for emergency procedures and how it impacts this moving and handling activity.

A legal pothole for care workers is knowing what they can and cannot do under first aid. This requires having a first aid certificate over and above the initial induction training. Effectiveness in first aid also depends on practice, practice and practice opportunities through frequent refresher training.

GDPR 2018 (DPA)

DPA was originally a 1998 Act that, in 2018[19], became the UK's implementation of the GDPR, which requires workers to follow strict rules called data protection principles.

Workers should realise that information such as the type of moving equipment they work with, the service user's reactions, actions and statements during the moving activity, and the contents of the care/handling plan or even what they observe about them are all confidential information that should not be discussed outside the workplace. Doing this will be a breach of the DPA.

---

[19] https://www.legislation.gov.uk/ukpga/2018/12/section/1/enacted

Organisations must ensure that their reporting procedure complies with GDPR, from data processing and usage to respecting the personal data of the service user who is the "data subject". All data is personal information belonging to the service user and cannot be used without permission. Organisations should also ensure registration and compliance with ICO regulations.

Domiciliary and care home contexts
All the above compliance issues anticipate both domiciliary and care homes and, in some cases, hospital settings. HSE recognises that it is easier for workers to carry out double-handed handling activity in a care home than in a domiciliary setting. It further recognises that working in care homes can also involve many other cleaning and maintenance tasks in places such as laundry, kitchens, and stores and, as such, risk more significant injuries because load or non-people handling is more prominent.[20]

Another difference between people handling in domiciliary and care home settings is that in the latter, relatives of the service user will not be in residence to assist as they would as carers in domiciliary settings; however, care home workers must respect relatives' choices and concerns for the service users.

Finally, workers in care homes will be used to a broader range of handling equipment than in domiciliary settings, which would be required to meet the needs of more users.

---

[20] HSE, 2014. *Health and Safety in Care Homes*. HSG22, p.17

Chapter Three
Holistic Approach to Moving and Handling

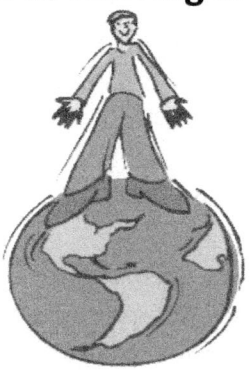

Why the Holistic and Compliance Approach?

'Moving and handling' is a CQC's knowledge and skills requirement as promoted by Skills for Care, Skills for Health, and NHS Health Education England in alignment with the CSTF. However, current training approaches to manual handling have not been working as they should.

MHOR 27 says that research "has found little evidence that training focusing primarily on handling techniques effectively promotes safer working and reduces injuries. The evidence suggests that techniques taught in training programmes often fail to be applied in the workplace".[21]

Most training relies more on workers' handling techniques without supporting them in addressing how to overcome "deficiencies such as unsuitable loads, bad working conditions or a lack of handling aids" that often accompany moving and

---

[21] https://www.hse.gov.uk/foi/internalops/ocs/300-399/313_5.htm

handling activities. Some of these deficiencies may be caused by a lack of in-depth and diverse understanding that influences the work environment, deficiencies that may require special skills and initiatives to correct or resolve. MHOR says these corrective or resolving skills and initiatives have failed to be applied in the workplace. The lack of appropriate skills will likely reflect incomplete or insufficient training and supporting resources such as training manuals and guides.

MHOR 28 further suggests, according to evidence, that injuries can be reduced by "multi-dimensional ergonomics interventions, involving the participation of workers and managers, and equipment. Coupled with training tailored to the person and specific task requirements." Training should be about "changing attitudes and behaviour and promoting risk awareness among workers and managers" that is "tailored to recipients' level of knowledge and understanding of the risks."[22]

The necessary question should, therefore, be: how should these workplace deficiencies and training failures be addressed? This can be achieved through a deeper holistic approach to moving and handling training. Only with a holistic approach can comprehensive knowledge and the right attitudes be brought into moving and handling activities.

A holistic approach to moving and handling people should anchor on the Code of Conduct that sets the standards expected of all adult social care workers and healthcare support workers in England,[23] detailed in the next section.

---

[22] *Ibid.*
[23] https://turboscholarship.com/94wals/what-should-be-included-in-the-code-of-conduct-bd9aae

Principles of Holistic Care

Holistic care requires broad thinking, the right attitude and empathy. Care workers should love what they do, be competent and always try to put themselves in the service user's shoes. This broad, comprehensive approach relies on three fundamental principles:
- Code of Conduct
- Recognising the values of the individual
- Giving respect and dignity to the individual

These principles and the subsequent components of holistic care anchor on attitude and empathy.

Attitude
According to the first Care Certificate standard, the role and responsibilities of a care worker rely on competence and the right attitude, which is significantly impacted by positive comprehensive induction training, workers' CPD and access to the correct information. A broad way of thinking and ethical work positively strengthen attitudes, and a positive attitude leads to effective care.

Empathy
This is defined as the "ability to understand the personal experience of the patient without bonding with them." Empathy is an "important communication skill" of emotional, cognitive, and behavioural attributes a health and social care worker should possess.[24] Those with these attributes elicit therapeutic change that makes service users feel safe.

---

[24] Moudatsou, Maria, et al., 2020, The Role of Empathy in Health and Social Care Professionals, MDPI, Basel.

Empathy in a professional context is similar and, in lay terms, used interchangeably with sympathy and compassion. Empathy helps guard against negative influences such as lack of respect and lateness to work. It should, therefore, be embedded in the organisation's training and work culture.

<u>Code of Conduct</u>
The Code by Skills for Care and Skills for Health is a non-compulsory outline of approved best practices on the behaviours and attitudes service users should expect from their care workers. A service user needs assurances that workers are expected to meet the requirements of their role, behave correctly and always do the right thing.

The Code is set out in three parts:
- The Code of Conduct for Care Workers
- The Code of Conduct for Employers
- Public awareness of the Code

Only the first two parts will be discussed.

The Code of Conduct for Care Workers
The Code of Conduct for Care Workers states that workers must: "Always make sure that" their "actions or omissions do not harm an individual's health or well-being", ensuring that they "never abuse, neglect, harm or exploit those who use health and care services, their carers, or…colleagues".[25]

The Code contains seven standards by which care workers are

---

[25] www.skillsforhealth.org.ul/code-of-conduct

held.[26] Workers must:
1. Be accountable by answering for their actions or omissions.
2. Promote and uphold service users' privacy, dignity, rights, health and well-being.
3. Collaborate with colleagues to deliver high-quality, safe, compassionate care and support.
4. Communicate openly and effectively to promote the safety and well-being of service users.
5. Respect service users' right to confidentiality.
6. Work to improve the quality of care and support through CPD.
7. Uphold and promote equality, diversity and inclusion.

The Care Certificate outlines the minimum knowledge that care workers require.

The Code of Conduct for Employers
This Code provides a clear set of standards for employers to:
1. Ensure the standards are met by their workers.
2. Check whether workers fulfil the requirements of their role, behave correctly, and always do the right thing.
3. Identify areas for employees' CPD.

Employers must provide workers with the proper support, training, and development to meet their obligations under the Code of Conduct.

They should agree on a Social Care Commitment with their workers to meet the minimum standards required in care work, provide education and learning, ensure a positive culture, and

---
[26] *Ibid.*

create a conducive working environment.

Recognising values

At the heart of person-centred care, according to the CQC, are six core values a care worker must always possess and work towards:

> **Care:** having someone's best interests at heart and doing the best to maintain or improve their well-being.
> **Compassion:** the ability to feel for someone and understand their situation.
> **Competence:** understanding what someone needs and having the knowledge and skills to provide it.
> **Communication:** listening carefully but also being able to speak and act in a way that the individual can understand.
> **Courage:** not fearing trying out new things or doing right.
> **Commitment:** dedication to providing care and support and understanding responsibility as a worker.

The service user also has values that must be recognised and respected, and the worker should allow them to be who and what they are or want to be. A worker must not impose their values on service users. The individual will most likely enjoy the moving and handling activity as they see the care worker as a professional and a person of respect.

Respect and dignity in equality & diversity at work

Manual handling is subject to care regulations, of which the Equality Act of 2010 is the mainstay of correct behaviour and attitude towards those receiving care.

Two crucial values when providing care and support are privacy and dignity. Privacy is giving someone space where and when needed, and dignity focuses on the individual's values.

The Act requires a set of actions for appreciation and compliance:[27]
- To avoid safeguarding concerns
- To research the values and needs of service users
- Provide person-centred care
- Respect service users' views, choices, and decisions
- Work with care and compassion
- Communicate directly with the individual whenever possible
- Respect confidentiality surrounding them
- Support them in making an informed choice
- Supporting their active participation
- Promote self-care
- Challenge discrimination on their behalf

Avoiding all situations of prejudice, such as discrimination, will help the care worker focus on the needs of the service user, meaning that what makes them different in terms of colour, age, sex, religion, and other protected characteristics should play no role in how they are cared for.

Components of Holistic Care

Self-care
People do this for themselves and their kin for physical, mental and general well-being. This ability to have control and care for oneself aids privacy and dignity and complements the care workers' activities in the workplace.

---

[27] https://www.legislation.gov.uk/ukpga/2010/15/contents

Skills for Care and Skills for Health have developed Common Core Principles for Self-Care. These principles aim to enable all those who work in health and social care to make personalised services a reality.[28]

At the heart of the self-care principle is the recognition that the service user is at the centre of the planning process and that they are best placed to understand their needs and how to meet them. This is more obvious in moving and handling as the service users are within the capacity expected to understand and contribute to their moving and handling activities. Those with the capacity should do the most difficult part of the moving activity rather than rely on the care worker to do it for them.

Communication
There is certainty that the care worker must briefly enter the service user's private space when moving and handling, and the individual must be comfortable with that brief or short-term, albeit "permitted intrusion". This is because they will be touched in many respects; however, it is the duty of the care worker to be professional about it and ensure that their handling is appropriate and explained. There are professional and non-professional ways of touching service users when moving and handling. This depends on communication skills.

Good communication skills create a trusting environment, enabling maximum support for well-being, while poor communication creates chaos and conflict. Good communication in care also involves informed consent. This is when the worker explains the moving procedure before the service user agrees. This allows them to ask questions and accept or deny an activity.

---

[28] www.skillsforcare.org.uk/Skills/Self-care/Self-care.aspx

Moving & Handling of People in Care Settings

Care workers should be able to employ several forms or types of communication, if necessary, such as verbal, sign language, braille, Makaton, facial expression, and eye contact, to calm the service user and earn their trust. Written communication skills aid effective reporting in moving and handling.

Workers must overcome communication barriers such as negative attitudes, limited use of technology, wrong body positioning, lateness to work, and not having enough rota time, thereby rushing the care activity. Other communication challenges are lack of confidentiality, stereotyping or respect for service users' privacy.

There should be frequent communication to involve the service user in moving activities to ensure the trust and cooperation of the individual. When speaking with the service user, the worker should try to be in front of them, making eye contact and speaking clearly.

The first time a worker is assigned to an individual, they should read the care/handling plan thoroughly and research the location to arrive on time, as this creates a good first impression. The service user should be greeted at the start, with the worker's ID shown. At the shift's end, it is polite also to greet them with a bye.

Finally, good communication is essential to gaining the individual's consent as it enables them to make informed decisions, which is at the heart of effective moving and handling care.

Confidentiality

Linked to communication is confidentiality. Records of daily handling activities must be kept appropriately and in the right places as the organisation requires.

Training on confidentiality, GDPR, privacy, and safety should be a part of induction and refresher training because service users appreciate those close to them who respect their space and are discrete. Information about the service user is their property and must not be shared with third parties not part of the official caring team. This may also mean workers should not gossip about service users within or outside the workplace. Neither should information about them be shared on social media.

Workers should pay attention to their observations of the service users and report accordingly. These important notes or records should not be in any place where they might be seen by someone else or stolen. They should be given to the care manager.

Reporting
Agreed ways of working in care are holistic because they cut across various levels of care. One such way of working is reporting incidents, accidents and concerns as the law requires. It is agreed that moving and handling is a regulated activity prone to health and safety challenges.

This is another reason why RIDDOR, explained in Chapter 2 above, is a crucial training topic. Employers and trainers are responsible for ensuring workers are competent enough to distinguish between incidents and accidents during moving and handling activities. Reporting under RIDDOR requires a moving and handling team always to include a "responsible person" or their designee who should submit the report under this legislation.

In moving and handling, falls, inadvertent harm or injuries caused by mistakes in handling equipment or manually can impact the overall care and well-being of the service user if not appropriately and quickly reported, enabling further care to be provided recovery and well-being.

Furthermore, what should also be reported by all workers regardless of RIDDOR status are concerns as these may have safeguarding consequences.

It is for these reasons that reporting is an essential holistic care factor.

Safeguarding

Safeguarding laws protect those we care for, especially those vulnerable to abuse, neglect, harm or exploitation. Complying with these laws promotes individuals' well-being and independence. Health and social care organisations are to deliver safe care and support. Every worker has a part to play in this process by constantly thinking of duty of care in terms of well-being and protecting them from abuse, neglect, harm or exploitation.

Abuses are significant elements of safeguarding and their forms are detailed in Chapter 2 above.

It is not difficult to see how the factors of principles of holistic care listed above relate to safeguarding, and it is as much about attitudes and behaviour as empathy and promoting awareness among workers and organisations. This makes safeguarding a holistic factor in care central to an individual's overall well-being, with particular concern for the proper conduct in every aspect of what constitutes care for a service user.

Fluids and nutrition

What we eat and drink affect human functionality, looks, and feelings. Good food and fluids aid in safe moving and handling because they improve human performance.

Good functionality makes cooperation possible and leads to positive outcomes in handling activities. Service users are more physically involved and can do the most difficult part of the moving action. This reduces care costs because the service user can migrate from double-handed to single-handed care.

Improved looks can also be important to the individual because of the self-esteem it promotes. This psychological boost often goes hand in hand with feelings. These are all important in manual handling, especially where personal care is involved.

Care workers should know about their balanced diet and good fluid habits for well-being and activity effectiveness. They should be able to work effectively with their colleagues who are responsible for the service user's nutrition. A properly and well-fed service user will be more alert and have a better physical capacity to assist in the physical elements of their moving and handling, which in turn eases the work of the care worker.

Fluids are essential for life, without which the body cannot carry out essential processes that enable it to function correctly. Fluids, especially water, digest food and enable the absorption of nutrients, allowing blood to circulate in the body. It also removes body wastes and maintains brain function. A well-hydrated service user perspires and cooperates better with moving and handling workers.

Moving and handling care workers should pay attention to signs of contamination in food and hazards that their service users may experience if they are also responsible for their nutrition. For instance, the care plan will indicate the individual's allergies and guide them if the service user has diabetes-related diseases.

Finally, adequate fluids and nutrition increase capacity and enable the prescribed medication to work correctly. This increased capacity to actively engage in moving and handling activities and other care activities makes fluids and nutrition perhaps the most significant components of holistic care.

Infections
Ignoring agreed ways of working on infection prevention and management poses health risks to care workers and service users, particularly during a moving and handling activity. A care worker should be trained to understand the broad categories and behaviours of germs that may affect the service users or themselves. These are:

- Bacteria
- Viruses
- Fungi
- Protozoa

They should also learn how to break the chains of the spread of infection. Preventing infection is about breaking the links in the chain to prevent spread, though some links are easier to break than others.

The COVID-19 pandemic is a cause for workers to pay extra attention to the risk of infections and strategies for their prevention in the workplace. The BMA confirmed this in its 2023 Report.

Preventing Infection
Steps to take in this process include the following:
- Wear protective clothing, gloves, and aprons (PPE).
- Wear disposable PPE only once and correctly. Discard it into a separate waste bag and tie it securely.
- Do not transfer moving and handling aids from one service user to another.
- Clean all aid equipment according to a Periodically following an agreed timetable.
- Maintain good hand hygiene after toileting and during food preparation.
- Keep all service users' washing items separate.
- Body waste (if a commode is used) must be flushed down the toilet with care. The commode, toilet and toilet seats must be disinfected.
- All infected bed linen, clothing, etc., must be identified, bagged, and washed separately.
- Follow the procedure for safe disposal of waste and safe management of laundry.
- Cover all open wounds with sticking plaster, etc.

Care/handling staff will be informed whether a service user has a contagious, infectious, or transmittable disease (if the information is available) if it is relevant to the job at hand and on a need-to-know basis.

Compliance with COSHH 2002
As a component in holistic care, this regulation-guided factor requires employers to control substances that are hazardous to

health. To reduce workers' exposure to hazardous substances, organisations can:[29]

- Find out what the health hazards are in the workplace.
- Decide how to prevent harm to health by undertaking a risk assessment.
- Provide control measures to reduce harm to health.
- Ensure that PPEs are correctly used.
- Keep all control measures in good working order.
- Provide appropriate information, instruction and training for employees and others.
- Provide health monitoring and surveillance in appropriate cases.
- Plan for emergencies.

Hazardous substances include dust, gases, fumes breathed in, or liquids, gels or powders that come into contact with the eyes or skin.

The significance of this factor is in risk prevention to have holistic well-being.

Emergency procedures in the workplace
In line with HSWA, a manual handling care worker is faced with certain situations that may impact the service they render or the well-being of their service users. Workers will probably be given some further training in these emergency procedures. Knowledge of and familiarisation with emergency procedures protect all care workers' hard work, the progress of the individual's well-being, and holistic care in general.

---

[29] https://www.hse.gov.uk/coshh/

Emergency Response and First Aid

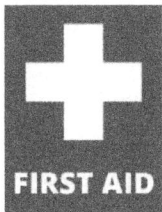

A care worker represents their organisation and must provide early warning of situations or problems that may cause concern. Not all emergencies will be life-threatening, but they require prompt and appropriate action.

In medical emergencies, guidelines must be followed, particularly knowing when to apply first aid before calling the emergency. In non-medical emergencies, care/handling workers should be aware of situations that may hamper handling, such as flooding, gas leakage, building damage, appliance malfunction, and equipment damage. Workers must assess the situation and give reassurance, using their knowledge and skills to alleviate it.

Fire Precaution

In the case of fire, knowledge of fire precautions is essential:
- Raise the alarm.

- If appropriate, assist the service user in leaving the premises if safe.
- Telephone 999, ask for the Fire Brigade - and give clear instructions about the location of the fire.
- If safe to do so, close windows and doors to prevent fire and smoke from spreading.
- Do not enter the building to collect personal belongings.

Gas Leakage

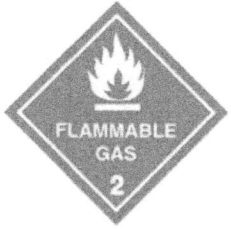

In this other emergency hazard, suppose they can smell gas or fumes; the worker should open windows to let it escape. They must turn off any fires or cookers and DO NOT LIGHT matches, candles, tapers, or cigarette lighters without putting themselves at risk.

Electricity and Appliances

It is necessary to read the care plan to see if any hazards or risks were found during the assessment. Electrical appliances should be checked before each use to ensure no deterioration has occurred since their last visit.

Depending on the service user's cognitive capacity, attention should be paid to electrical components to decide whether they could be covered with plastic plugs. All concerns should be reported immediately to the care manager.

Caring in a Holistic Way

The handling workers should understand that moving and handling activities cannot be exercised in isolation from other care components.

They should know about the connectivity and inter-relatedness as well as the boundaries of each of these components, and only then can they truly provide sustainable handling care.

Finally, training and organisational resources should be invested in a holistic rather than a singular approach to care. What will be the use to a service user in the long run if they are well fed but cannot trust their environment due to poor communication or an infection infecting them due to a worker's negligence?

Proper handling care is where the individual is engaged, hoping for better involvement, comfort, and a better and independent future.

Moving & Handling of People in Care Settings

Chapter Four
Human Back, Injuries and Diseases

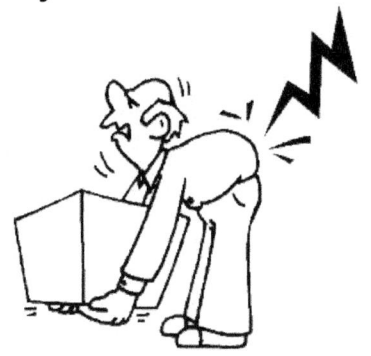

The Biomechanics of Human Movement and the Back

Biomechanics
Biomechanics is all about working the body in the most efficient and least stressful way, of which the stability of the human support base is an intrinsic part. Biomechanics recognises that the human support base consists of the feet and the area between them, requiring the stability of keeping up the line of gravity within the support base.

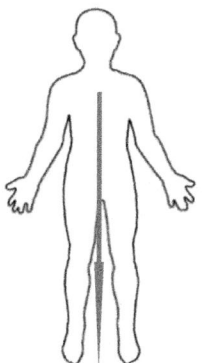

The line of gravity is the vertical direction down to the floor from the centre of gravity. Total body mass is concentrated within this centre of gravity, and the body has to alter its dimensions depending on how external factors impact its centre of gravity.

When this dimension is altered, the line is forced to move from the centre of gravity to fall outside the base, causing instability and strain to the back. Hence, body parts partaking in these dynamics should be as short as possible. Arms should bend at the right angle; legs kept as short as possible, knees bent, feet

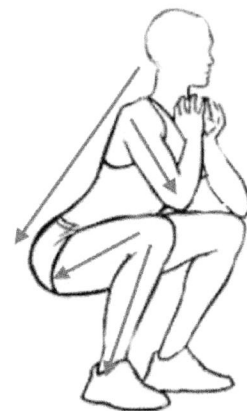

slightly apart, thus widening so that the base is firm and the line of gravity within the base of support is balanced.

Purpose of the back
The purpose of the back is to complete a person. It is vital in day-to-day living and crucial to walking, standing, playing, sitting, sleeping, working, and enjoying. Work is lifting, bending, and, indeed, any human activity.

Human torso
The human torso houses vital human organs. The front of the torso is from the chest and the abdomen. The back is the

posterior area rising from the top of the buttocks to the back of the neck. The organs include the vertebral column, the backbone or the spine.

Vertebral column

The vertebral column, which has the shape of an elongated 'S', is a cavity that encases the spinal canal, protecting the spinal cord.

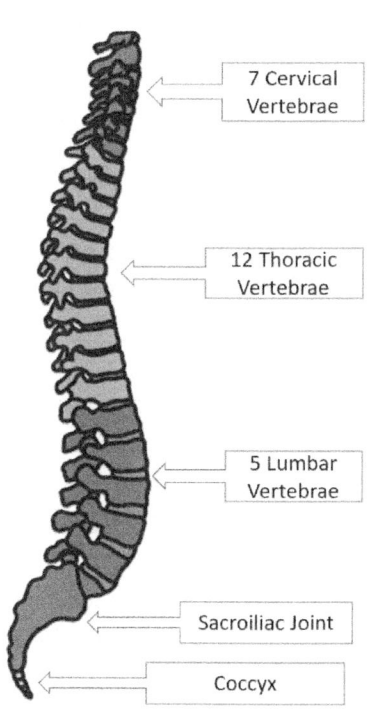

The natural "S" curves balances the body and keeps the head up.

If the "S" shape is altered then the discs are pressured, ligaments are strained and muscles may be pulled

- 7 Cervical Vertebrae
- 12 Thoracic Vertebrae
- 5 Lumbar Vertebrae
- Sacroiliac Joint
- Coccyx

The "S" shape can be altered through:
- Slouching
- Poor posturing
- Bad/sudden movement, such as jerking
- Bad positioning
- Excessive/repetitive straining movements

Structure of the back/components

The components of the back include:
- Spine
- Facet Joints
- Intervertebral discs
- Muscles
- Ligaments
- Spinal cord
- Spinal Nerves

Spine: its 33 bones are known as vertebrae, though it consists of other parts such as joints, discs, soft tissues, nerves and the spinal cord. The upper 24 bones (cervical, thoracic and lumbar) are separated by discs that act as cushions in the biomechanics. The spine supports the body in its activities.

Facet Joints link the vertebrae together, stabilising and protecting the spine from excessive shear rotational and flexion forces and movement. In effect, they limit awkward movements such as bending and twisting.

Intervertebral Discs are the structures located between adjacent vertebrae of the spine. Each disc consists of a tough outer layer called the *annulus fibrosus* and the gel-like centre called the *nucleus pulposus*.[30] These can degenerate over time. The functions of intervertebral discs are:[31]
- Shock absorption

---

[30] https://jointspinerehab.com/understanding-herniated-discs-causes-symptoms-and-diagnosis/
[31] *https://www.spineinfo.com*

- Load-bearing
- Flexibility and mobility
- Spacing of vertebrae
- Nutrient supply

Muscles are bands of fibrous tissues that contract together to produce movement or a force that maintains the position of parts of the body. Numbering up to 400, muscles produce motion in all directions while supporting the spine in the upright position to produce and control movement.

Muscles are of three types:[32]
1. **The Skeletal muscle** consisting of striated tissues attached to the skeleton that apply force to bones and joints via contraction to create movement.
2. **The Cardiac muscle** is an involuntary striated type found in the wall of the heart.
3. **The Smooth muscle** is the non-striated type found within the arteries, veins, reproductive gastrointestinal and respiratory tract, bladder, uterus, and eye.

In moving and handling, attention should be paid to the following muscle locations in the body:
        Shoulder Girdle
        Shoulder Joint
        Elbow Joint
        Wrist and Hand
        Thigh & Knee

---
[32] https://graphdiagram.com/types-of-muscle/

Hip and Groin
Lower Leg and Ankle
Neck and Back

Ligaments, like muscles, are short, dense and tough bands of fibrous connective tissues that connect two bones or cartilages or hold together a joint that adds to the spine's stability. They do not contract like muscles but are passive.

Spinal Cord is a forty-five-centimetre-long central nervous system tissue part about a half-inch thick linking the brain stem to the lumbar region, supplying nerves and transmitting and receiving information within the body. It directs all activities below the neck level, passing down through the middle of the spinal column in the spinal canal.

The cord must be protected within the spinal canal. It is, therefore, easy to see that damage to the spine affecting the spinal cord would affect a person severely.

Spinal Nerves branch off at each level of the vertebral column, carrying nerve impulses (sensory and motor) to and from the various body structures, particularly between the brain and other body parts. They are in pairs of 31.

Damage to the spine
Damage to the spine through slouching, poor posturing, stress, bad/sudden movement or positioning or excessive or repetitive straining movements could alter the vertebral column 'S' shape or and/or expose the spinal cord, which may protrude from its

Its encasement causes nerve traps or damage, affecting the transmission of information around the body or movement.

A closer look at a section of the spine below shows how this can happen.

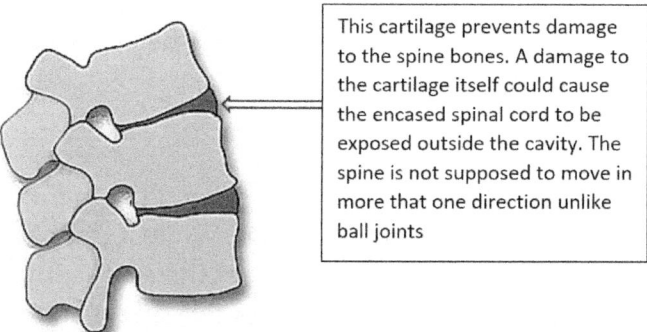

This cartilage prevents damage to the spine bones. A damage to the cartilage itself could cause the encased spinal cord to be exposed outside the cavity. The spine is not supposed to move in more that one direction unlike ball joints

MSDs

Manual handling injuries are mostly part of a wider group of musculoskeletal disorders known as MSDs. The term covers injuries, damages or disorders of the joints or other upper/lower limb tissues. MSDs can result from care handling work activities or even illnesses or diseases unrelated to work.

Work-related MSDs, including manual handling injuries, are the UK's most common type of occupational ill health. Even where MSDs cannot be prevented, a lot can be done to minimise their impacts, such as early reporting of symptoms, proper treatment and suitable rehabilitation.

The symptoms of MSDs
These are:
- Paralysis
- Loss of or altered sensation affecting temperature, bowel, or bladder
- Spasms
- Difficulty breathing or coughing
- Pain or stinging sensation may be caused by damage to the nerve

Back pain
Back pain is a common medical condition and the second most common type in adults after headaches. While it can have many causes, back pain tends to get better, yet the most common cause of back pain is pulled muscle strain. Workers should pay early attention to pain in the back area, and rest should be taken. A mental review of work habits, such as bad posturing, should also be undertaken.

Spinal cord injury
Damaging parts of the nerves or spinal cord may cause permanent changes in sensation, strength and other body functionality below the injury site. This may impact one's mental, psychological and social well-being.

"A spinal cord injury can be complete or incomplete. This depends on the severity of the injury. It is complete if all feelings (sensory) and all ability to control movement (motor function) are lost below the spinal cord injury;" it is incomplete if there are still some feelings or control movement below the affected area.[33]

If paralysis occurs due to the injury, this will be referred to as tetraplegia or quadriplegia if arms, hands, trunk, legs and pelvic organs are all affected. If, however, the resulting paralysis may affect all or part of the legs, trunk, and pelvic organs, it is known as paraplegia.

Workers should be alert to the following emergency signs and symptoms of spinal cord injuries, especially after an accident, which can be:[34]
- Difficulty with balance and walking
- Twisted neck or back
- Changes to sensation such as inability to feel the heat and cold or loss of sense of touch
- Breathing difficulty, coughing or lung secretions clearing
- "Extreme back pain or pressure in the neck, head or back
- Weakness, incoordination or paralysis in any part of the body
- Numbness, tingling or loss of sensation in the hands, fingers, feet or toes
- Loss of bladder or bowel control."[35]

Other causes of spinal cord injuries and trauma are:
- Sporting accidents
- Violent events such as stabbing
- Vascular disorders

---

[33] https://www.mayoclinic.org/diseases-conditions/spinal-cord-injury/symptoms-causes/syc-20377890
[34] https://spinalcordinjuryzone.com/info/7335/signs-and-symptoms-of-sci
[35] *Ibid.*

- Tumours
- Infectious conditions
- Developmental disorders
- Spondylosis
- Vertebral fractures

Emergency procedure in back/neck injury
If it is suspected that someone has a back or neck injury:
- Do not move them to avoid permanent paralysis or other serious complications
- Call the emergency
- Keep the individual still
- "Place heavy towels on both sides of the neck or hold the head and neck to prevent them from moving until emergency care arrives
- Provide basic first aid in case of bleeding or unresponsiveness."[36]

Other Injuries and accidents in the workplace and types
Accidents are more straightforward causes of injuries when moving people, and legislation exists to help ensure that all activities have the best practices to reduce the risk of injury to the care worker and the service user.

Types
Bruising
Crushed fingers or toes
Fractures
Cuts and grazes
Strains and sprains dislocation
Soft tissue damage

---
[36] https://ledezmalawfirm.com/injuries/spine-injuries/

Back acute pain
Chronic Herniated disc
Hernia
Spina bifida
Scoliosis

Steps to take if an individual is injured
1. Identify the injury type.
2. Get help.
3. Do not move the person unless in further danger, such as a fire threat.
4. Reassure the individual by telling them about the moving plan.
5. Employ the proper techniques.
6. Protect the back always.
7. Use the right equipment on which workers have been trained.
8. Be aware of children or other vulnerable people in the vicinity.

Illnesses and Disability Impacting Moving and Handling

Physical illnesses
Other than back-related injuries, moving and handling workers should be aware that physical illnesses can pose severe challenges to moving and handling activities.

Service users currently being treated for physical ailments must be made comfortable by workers before moving and handling activity commences. They may encounter illnesses like arthritis, angina, asthma, bronchitis, brittle bones, cancer, diabetes, emphysema, rheumatism, and sight loss.

Mental illnesses

As explained in Chapter Two above on mental capacity, a moving and handling worker may face the challenges of those who can no longer make their own decisions because they have a condition that can affect their cognitive abilities. Workers must follow MCA 2005 requirements, as those with these conditions are still required to make informed decisions or choices.

Workers should be able to recognise the signs and symptoms of mental health conditions and episodes that could cause abrupt termination or delays in moving and handling activities. These signs and symptoms may include:

- Dementia
- Manic depression
- Schizophrenia
- Anxiety
- Phobia
- Depression
- Loneliness
- Isolation

The above conditions may be more associated with elderly service users, but not always.

Workers should look for signs of negativity, hopelessness, sadness, or even aggression and frustration accompanying the above signs, particularly depression. In the case of dementia, there may be signs of anger, frustration, forgetfulness or hallucination. These are very complex situations, and workers will do well not to stereotype the individual.

Workers should exercise patience, sympathy, and empathy because they may face challenges of memory complications often found in dementia where a service user's memories may play up, for instance, persistently recalling things that happened a long time ago or forgetting that they just had meals or personal care. These sometimes affect their willingness or ability to cooperate with workers, and they may not always be able to do the most difficult part of their moving and handling activity.

Workers, in turn, must look after their physical and mental health because these conditions may impact them.

Children and young persons

Working with children and young people in moving and handling is much the same as working with adults. Their care plan would have been agreed upon with the organisation's client by a parent, guardian relative, or local authority.

The areas of difference between adults and young people are in applying the legislation, particularly compliance with *Safeguarding Disabled Children and Young People - Inter-agency Practice Guidance.*

Laws for protecting young people are set out in MHSWR Regulations 19. According to the law, children are guided by the paramountcy principle that deems them more vulnerable than adults. Additional or enhanced DBS background checks and further workers' training may be required. There may also be different company policies and procedures in place.

The law recognises young people as those below 18 years of age who need protection from risks because of their supposed lack of experience, awareness of existing or potential risks, and lack of "full maturity".[37] This may make working within a care setting more difficult for young people. Workers should look out for those pranks or what some may deem naughty behaviour from them, as some may be prone to playing pranks on workers.

Employers should be aware of the need not to employ children illegally. When qualified young persons are in the workplace, they should not be given tasks beyond their physical or psychological capacity or tasks that will expose their insufficient attention to safety or lack of experience or training. They should always be under supervision.

In addition to the CQC carrying out statutory inspections of care facilities or workplaces, the OFSTED may also oversee policies and procedures. See the section on training in Chapter Seven below for a better understanding of how to deal with children and young people.

Learning disability
Closely with children and young people is understanding the care for those with learning disabilities.

Those with learning disabilities may also present challenges such as those faced by workers in MCA environments. Most of those cognitively impacted by trauma, diseases or hereditary may be slow at learning, affecting their emotional and social development.

It should be considered that adults with some types of mental health conditions may also fall into this category. Moving and

---

[37] MHSWR Regulations 19

handling workers' success in the above situations will depend significantly on their training and communication skills.

Some statistics and costs of injuries
1. About 30% of all back injuries are attributed to slips, trips, or falls.
2. About 22% are attributed to lifting/handling.
3. About 10% are struck by objects, whilst about 7% fall from heights.
4. Each year, there are around 500,000 work-related back illnesses.

Cost of injuries to the economy
- Days lost
- Staff replacement costs
- Reduced efficiencies
- Increased insurance premium
- Disruption of work schedules
- Increased litigations against employers

Cost of injuries to moving and handling care worker
- Back or other musculoskeletal injuries
- Loss of income
- Back problems later in life

Cost of workers' injuries to the organisation
- Loss of experienced staff
- Changes to work schedules
- Increased workload
- Loss of continuity of care
- Commercial losses

By 2020, MSDs will account for about 30% of GP consultations in England. They are estimated to cost the NHS £4.76 billion each year.[38]

Concerning NHS staff, the National Health Executive, NHE, claims that UK taxpayers are footing £400 million annually for staff who have injured their backs at work. This total includes staff sickness, absence, and wasted training. The other consequence is that each year, more than 80,000 nurses sustain back injuries while 3,600 healthcare workers are forced into early retirement.[39]

In 2020, HSE said that the cost of workplace injury was £18.8b. In 2022, 1.8 million working people suffered from a work-related illness, of which 477,000 workers had a work-related musculoskeletal disorder. 36.8 million working days are lost due to work-related illnesses and workplace injuries.[40]

---

[38] Manchester Metropolitan University: "Back pain costs the NHS nearly £5 billion, physiotherapists have an ever-increasing role to play in relieving strain on services" December 2020. https:// www.mmu.ac.uk/news-and-vents/news/story/?id=13353
[39] https://www.nationalhealthexecutive.com/News/huge-cost-of-back-injuries-to-the-nhs
[40] *Ibid.*

Chapter Five
Manual Handling of Objects

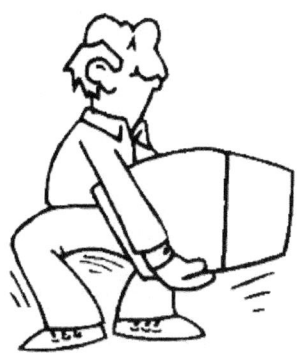

Objects Handling Activities and Principles

Manual handling activities
Activities associated with handling inanimate objects are:
- Pulling
- Pushing
- Carrying
- Unloading
- Lifting
- Lowering
- Team Lift
- Awkward / Special Objects Lift
- Overhead Lift - Lift or lowering to/from a high place
- Squat Lift

Handling inanimate objects is a care support activity defined in health and social care, manual handling legislation, and the Code of Conduct. Care workers must carry out these activities with or without notice in domiciliary and care home settings. Objects

that tend to be handled in the workplace may include:**[41]
- Grocery shopping bags
- Deliveries and boxes
- Furniture relocation, such as chairs or small desks
- Moving equipment, etc

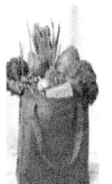 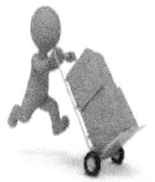 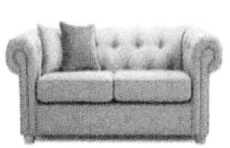 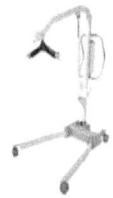

Handling inanimate objects in the workplace is also a regulated care support activity because of the possible health and safety risks to the workers and their service users. As legislation affirms, manual handling focuses on avoiding injury to the care worker and others.

Manual handling guidelines
MHOR sets out the hierarchy of measures for <u>*organisations*</u> to follow to prevent and manage the risks from hazardous manual handling:
1. **Avoid** hazardous manual handling operations as reasonably practicable as possible.
2. **Assess** the risk of injury to workers from hazardous manual handling that cannot be avoided.

---

[41] *** To avoid injury, shopping bags, for instance, should not be carried if too heavy in one bag but should be distributed in two bags evenly and carry one in each hand. Moving some of the home furniture around may require the permission of the care manager, except those for daily use.*

3. **Reduce** the risk of injury to workers from hazardous manual handling as low as reasonably practicable.
4. **Review** Risk Assessments when changes occur or are no longer valid.

MHOR also sets out the duty of <u>workers</u>. It says that for their health and safety, they should:
1. Follow systems of work in place.
2. Use properly any equipment provided.
3. Cooperate with the organisations on health and safety matters.
4. Inform the organisation if things change or they identify hazardous handling activities.
5. Ensure that their activities do not put others at risk.

<u>Principles and techniques of manual handling of inanimate objects</u>

There are several ways to control manual handling risks. The best practice is to design activity processes that first avoid handling and, if unavoidable, minimise risks posed.

During a manual handling activity, the following principles must always be adhered to:
1. Is handling necessary or avoidable?
2. Examining the object to –
    a. Determine its weight by looking for any information/advice label.
    b. Look for sharp edges or awkward parts.
    c. Look for uneven stability or unequal distribution.
3. Planning –
    a. Decide if:

i. Manual handling is necessary, or
ii. If equipment is required, or
iii. More the activity requires more than one person or
iv. If the load needs to be divided into smaller parts:
- Employing a mechanical device.
- Wearing the right equipment if required.
- Getting help if necessary.

b. Before lifting, ensure the entire path is safe and free from potential physical, chemical or biological hazards.

4. Body Positioning –
   a. The body's centre of gravity must be stable, feet apart, firmly on the ground and no wider than the hips. This is called the *dynamic stable base*.
   b. This is followed by bending the knees to a squat position, avoiding bending the back, and leaning forward to avoid stress on the lower back.
   c. The next position before lift-off is firm and secure grip on the load, keeping the back upright and straightening the legs.

(Lifter can also adopt a static position: feet firmly apart with one leg slightly forward for support).

5. Picking and moving with the object –
   a. Upward, using the leg muscles to lift the object.
   b. Tense the back and stomach muscles.
   c. Keeping the object close to the body with the back upright.

Moving & Handling of People in Care Settings

6. Proceeding with –
    a. A steady, firm grip:
       Keeping head and spine upright
    b. Walking with feet in the direction of the load destination, avoiding twisting, stooping or bending.
    c. To turn and move the feet is better than twisting and lifting simultaneously.
        i. Shoulders should level and face in the same direction as the hips.
        ii. Determine if there will be rest stops
7. Placing the object in the destination –
    a. Lowering the load.
    b. Keeping a good posture.
    c. Bending the knees using leg muscles.
    d. Positioning the object securely.

<u>Other types of manual lift</u>

Individual Manual Lifts (1)

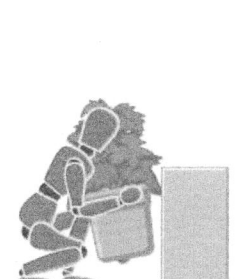 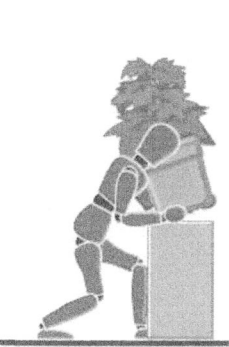 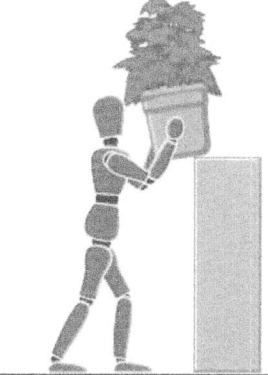

Individual Manual Lifts (2)

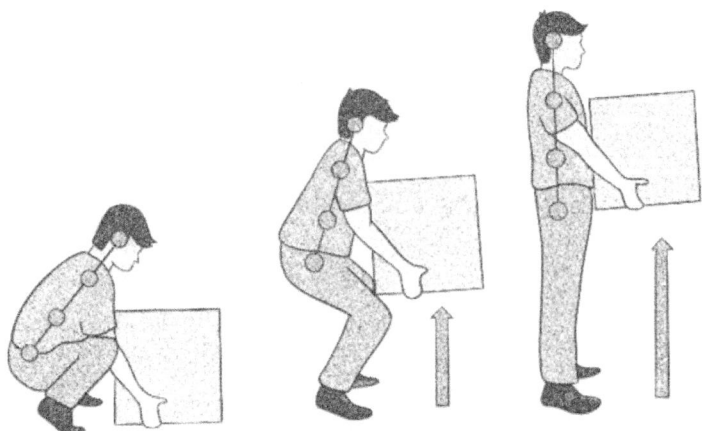

Team Manual Lifts

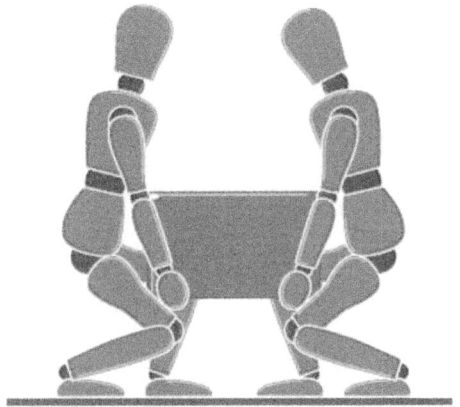

Other safety guidelines

HSE Lifting and Lowering risk filters[42]
Filter values for handling operations when seated:

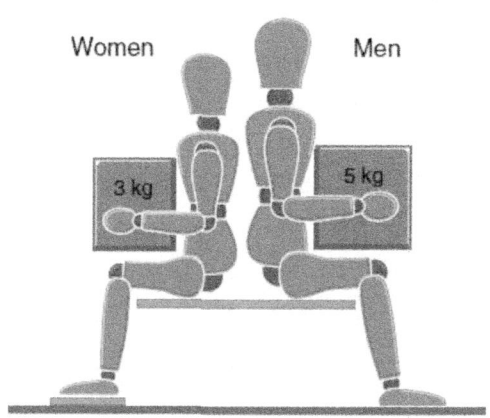

HSE Lifting and Lowering risk filters[43]

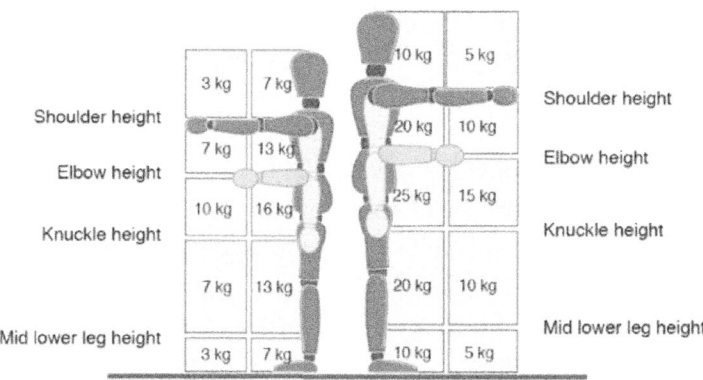

Workers should consider the zone of height, load and maximum weight. Use a smaller weight in each zone if the hand extends beyond the zone close to the body.

---

[42] https://www.hse.gov.uk/msd/manual-handling-risk-filters.htm
[43] *Source: HSE Manual handling*

Types of Risk Assessment in Moving and Handling

MHSWR requires organisations to assess workers' health and safety risks, and where hazardous manual handling of loads is identified, they should comply with the MHOR tools below:

A. Manual Handling Assessment Charts (MAC) tool

HSE developed a MAC tool aimed at employers, health and safety managers and inspectors to identify high-risk manual handling. MAC assesses handling's most common risk factors.

It assesses:
1. Lifting operations.
2. Carrying operations.
3. Team handling operations.

MAC is not appropriate for:
1. Operations involving pushing and pulling.
2. Assessing people handling.
3. Assessing workplace risks associated with upper limb disorders.

How to complete a MAC assessment:[44]
1. Identify the tasks to assess.
2. Choose hard tasks that employees complain about.
3. Consult employees about the most challenging tasks.
4. Observe the task and ensure looking at how it is usually done.
5. "Follow the appropriate assessment guide and flow chart to determine each factor's risk level.
6. Look for ways to modify the task to reduce the red

---

[44] https://www.hse.gov.uk/msd/mac/tips.htm

risk factors to amber or green and to reduce amber risk factors to green.
7. Prioritise action by addressing the task with the highest total score first".

The total scores do not relate to specific action levels.

B. Risk Assessment of Pushing and Pulling (RAPP) tool

"RAPP tool is designed to help assess the key risks in manual pushing and pulling operations involving whole-body effort". It should be used alongside the MAC tool.

It is aimed at those responsible for health and safety in workplaces, helping to identify high-risk pushing and pulling activities whilst checking the effectiveness of any risk-reduction measures.

RAPP recognises two types of pulling and pushing operations of moving:
1. Loads on wheeled equipment, such as hand trolleys.
2. Loads without wheels requiring actions such as dragging/sliding

In RAPP, an associated sliding flow chart is also provided as an assessment guide, and a score sheet is provided to give an overview of the risk factors and assessment process.

How to complete the RAPP assessment:
1. Observe and consult workers on the work activity to note work practice.
2. Consider the 'worst-case scenario'.
3. Select the appropriate assessment (i.e. pushing and pulling wheeled or non-wheeled equipment, for instance).

4. Follow the appropriate flow chart and assessment guide to determine the risk level for each risk factor. (For risk levels, see HOP6, *The guide to the handling of people: A systems approach*).

C. Full risk assessment
It is advised to use the HSE's guidance booklet L23 *Manual Handling. Manual Handling Operations Regulations 1992: Guidance on Regulations* for full risk assessment. This relates to both inanimate and people handling.

Assessing the risks
Where risks from hazardous manual handling in the workplace cannot be avoided, a manual handling risk assessment is required to manage these risks. It is vital to involve the workforce in the risk assessment process.

Consideration for Risk Assessment:
1. The **T**ask
2. **I**ndividual capacity
3. The **L**oad
4. The **E**nvironment

Consider the individual requirements of workers who may be at risk, such as pregnancy, disability, recently injured, inexperienced new workers, young or temporary workers, older workers, contractors, migrant workers who may not have English as their first language or other psychosocial risk factors.

Risks and controls in manual handling (objects and people)
Risks Associated with the TASKS
The tasks

Do they involve:
1. Holding loads away from the body?
2. Twisting, stooping or reaching upwards?
3. Large vertical movement?
4. Long carrying distances?
5. Strenuous pushing or pulling?
6. Repetitive handling?
7. Risk of sudden movement of loads?
8. Insufficient rest or recovery time?
9. A work rate imposed by a process?

Ways of reducing the risk of injury
Can the worker:
1. Use a lifting aid?
2. Change workplace layout to improve efficiency?
3. Reduce the amount of twisting and stooping?
4. Avoid lifting from floor level or above shoulder height, especially heavy loads?
5. Reduce carrying distances?
6. Use powered handling devices to eliminate pushing and pulling?
7. Avoid repetitive handling?
8. Take steps to reduce fatigue?

Risks Associated with INDIVIDUAL CAPACITY
The Individual (Considering the worker's capacity)
Does the job:
1. Require unusual capability, e.g. above average strength or agility? Does the worker have the strength to do it?
2. Pose a risk to those with a health problem or learning/physical disability? Is the worker healthy enough?
3. Pose a risk to new or expectant mothers?

4. Pose a risk to new or young workers?
5. Call for special information or training?

Ways of reducing the risk of injury
Can the organisation/worker:
1. Consider the design of the task?
2. Pay particular attention to those who have a physical weakness?
3. Take extra care of new or expectant mothers and new/young workers?
4. Give workers more information, e.g. about the range of tasks?
5. Provide more training?

Risks Associated with LOAD
The loads
Are they:
1. Heavy or bulky?
2. Difficult to grasp?
3. Unstable or likely to move unpredictably?
4. Harmful, e.g. sharp or hot?
5. Awkwardly stacked?
6. Is it too large for the handler to see over?

Ways of reducing the risk of injury
Can the worker make the load:
1. Lighter or less bulky?
2. Easier to grasp?
3. More stable?
4. Less harmful?
5. Evenly stacked?
6. Split into smaller packages?

Risks Associated with the ENVIRONMENT
In the working environment
Are there:

1. Restrictions on posture?
2. Bumpy, obstructed or slippery floors?
3. Variations in floor levels?
4. Hot/cold/humid conditions?
5. Gusts of wind or other strong air movements?
6. Poor lighting conditions?
7. Restrictions on movements from clothes or personal protective equipment (PPE)?

Ways of reducing the risk of injury
Can the worker:
1. Remove obstructions to free movement?
2. Provide better flooring and/or slip-resistant footwear?
3. Avoid steps, stairs and steep ramps?
4. Prevent extremes of hot and cold?
5. Improve ventilation?
6. Improve lighting?
7. Provide suitable protective clothing or PPE that is less restrictive?

PARTICULAR Risks Associated with HANDLING AIDS & EQUIPMENT
Handling aids and equipment
Considerations by the Organisation:
1. Is the device the correct type for the job?
2. Is it well maintained and LOLER/PUWER certified?
3. Are the device's handles, wheels, brakes, and battery in good condition?

Ways of reducing the risk of injury
Can the organisation:
1. Provide equipment that is more suitable for the task?
2. Carry out statutory/preventive maintenance?
3. Provide appropriate training on specific equipment?

PARTICULAR Risks Associated with WORK ORGANISATION FACTORS

Work organisation factors
Considerations by the Organisation:
1. The repetitiveness of the work?
2. Do workers feel the demands of the work are excessive?
3. Do workers have little control of the work and Working methods?
4. Is there poor communication between managers and workers?

Ways of reducing the risk of injury
1. Changing tasks amongst workers to increase variety.
2. Make more use of workers' skills.
3. Make workloads and deadlines more achievable.
4. Involve workers in decisions.
5. Encourage good communication and teamwork.
6. Provide better training and information.

<u>Factors influencing risk reduction</u>
Risks can be reduced by understanding the following factors:
1. **Type of load** being lifted, its weight, shape and composition;
2. **Risk associated with a load** falling, moving, breaking up, or striking a person or object and the consequences;
3. **Risk of the lifting equipment** striking a person or an object and the consequences;
4. **Risk of the failure of lifting equipment** or falling over while in use, and the consequences and
5. **Risk of damage to the lifting equipment** that could fail.

Chapter Six
Moving and Handling of People

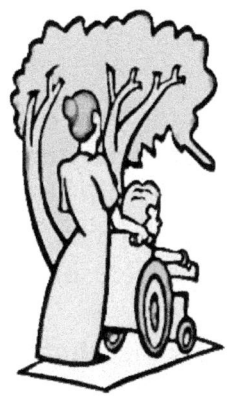

Moving and Handling of People's Activities

General activities associated with people's moving and handling that organisations should submit to risk assessments are:
- Getting in or out of bed
- Hoisting
- Lifting
- Moving in wheelchairs
- Moving up and down stairs
- Personal care, including bathing, toileting and dressing
- Standing
- Sitting up in bed or chair
- Team Lifting
- Transfers in all the above situations and into/from vehicles
- Turning over in bed
- Walking

The principles of moving and handling people

While manual handling of objects differs from moving and handling of people, the similarities of their respective principles lie in the premise that the handling activities may be avoidable.

There are two differences in these respective principles of avoidability, however. First is the question of the well-being and needs of the service user, which is not present in the case of manual handling of objects. The second difference is the risk of injury to the service user and the care worker.

In moving and handling people, there are the following essential principles:
1. Always try to avoid manual handling.
2. The focus of the task is to avoid injury to the care worker and the service user.
3. A risk assessment or control of risks is continuous.
4. The service user is expected to do the most difficult activity while moving.
5. Where the service user cannot temporarily or permanently do the most difficult task, an assessment should be made if handling them would require two or more care workers or use equipment safe enough for one person to handle.
6. If several workers are involved, a collective strategy should be agreed.
7. Care workers must work according to guidelines and the individual's handling plan.
8. The service user must be handled with dignity and respect.
9. Keep records of activities, observations, incidents, and incidents in the RIDDOR way.

Moving & Handling of People in Care Settings

Strategy for moving and handling people
1. Follow the care and handling plan.
2. Plan the activity:
    a. Consider if moving and handling is necessary. Improvement in the service user's condition may inform this, but the decision is left to the service user and care manager.
    b. Agree with the organisation's manager if the situation changes. (Think individual, environment or equipment).
    c. Discuss with other care workers and agree to a plan.
    d. Discuss the agreed plan with the service user.
3. Ensure service user is supported in a holistic way, including:
    a. That they have taken their meal and fluid.
    b. That they have taken their medication if required before handling.
    c. That they are willing and ready to participate in the activity.
4. Follow practical methods learnt and agreed upon by the organisation and the aids manufacturer's instructions.
5. Observe or listen to the service user's discomfort and give them confidence by reassuring them if they are agitated during the moving activity.

Common moving and handling situations
Assuring the individual
It is necessary that in all handling situations, communication with service users gives some assurance.

Assisting mobility: Level Walking

Assess the walking capability of the service user before walking with them.

The care worker should position themself on the individual's weaker side, supporting them with one hand around them and asking them to clasp their nearer hand and place it in the palm of the care worker, avoiding a heavy palm grasp and walking

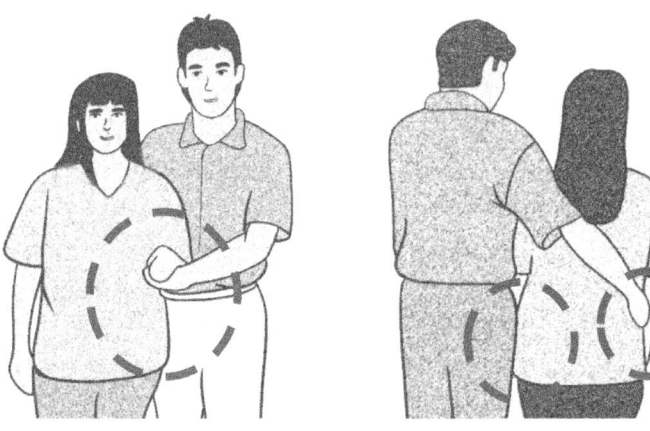

slowly, their hips touching and guiding the service user.

Assisting mobility: Stairs Walking

Walking up and down the stairs is a challenge without a stairlift.

In walking up the stairs, the care worker should stand two steps below the individual, holding the bannister and steadying themselves by putting one hand on the service user's hip.

Walking downstairs, the same principle applies when standing two steps below the service user but facing them, placing a hand

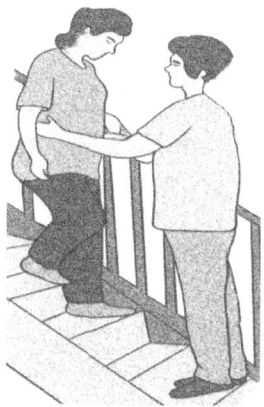

on their hip, guiding them slowly, and keeping both feet on the same step.

Stairlift

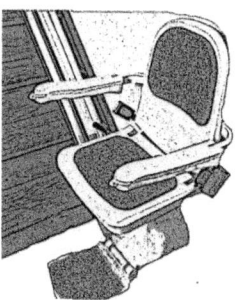

Stairlifts may be a solution to stairwalking and have reduced the risks involved in this activity.

Moving in and out of bed
A bed-bound service user would need to be turned in and out of bed for comfort and to avoid bed soreness; otherwise, it is necessary to move service users out of bed for general and physical well-being.

They will need to sit in bed and transfer to the commode, the bath, chair, wheelchair, etc. These should be done with utmost care, respect and support of necessary aids and equipment. This activity will also probably require a double-handed approach if the individual cannot do the most difficult part of the activity.
(For more information, see the section on sliding sheets below.)

Sitting-to-standing
Standing from a bed, chair, wheelchair, commode, or any other device is a core activity a care worker should support the service users with, depending on their capacity.

Commonly, a service user who cannot help do the most difficult part of getting up may not be able to stand alone for long. An example of this difficult part expected of a service user from standing is putting both hands on a seat or wheelchair handle and lifting themselves with strength.

To do this, the following suggestions would be necessary:
- Encourage them to shuffle/rock to the front edge of the seat.
- Their feet are firm on the floor.
- Their weight forwards.
- Their nose over toes
- Arms pushing on fixed support such as the seat handle.
- They may also place their hand on the workers' hands for a push-up.
- Do not push them up on walking aids such as the Zimmer frame or walking stick.

A handling belt may provide the solution for this situation.

Standing-to-sitting: repositioning in a chair

Repositioning a service user to where they were previously moved from is a particular task facing handling workers. As in sitting-to-standing above, the service user is still expected to do the most difficult part of sitting from standing, for example, being able to put one or both hands on a chair handle and steady themselves to sit with minimal support from the workers.

Repositioning may be initially from a bed, commode, or any other device before the service user stands up. This also assumes the capacity to walk even if assisted.

- Ensure the chair is correctly positioned and sturdy.
- Upon reaching the chair, they should turn around with the chair behind them.
- They should be able to use at least one arm to lower themself into the chair.
- With an assist to the side, they can use one arm to hold on to the chair armrest while placing a weaker arm on the worker's palm.
- Workers must kneel beside the service user and lower them into the chair.

Once seated, they should shuffle/rock themselves back in the chair.

If in doubt, hoist them. This activity may be double-handed if a handling belt or hoist is required.

Special moving and handling situations
Assisting mobility: Impaired vision
Those with impaired vision are usually happy being independent. However, when support is needed, the care worker should either cup their hand under the service user's elbow or allow them to take the care worker's arm. They should

walk at the service user's side or close enough to maintain contact and warn of hazards ahead of the route.

Lifting off the Floor
A service user should be lifted off the floor with a hoist and sling if they cannot support themself in getting off the floor. Lifting off the floor without lifting equipment requires much practice during training.

This activity presumes that the service user can do the most difficult lifting. These difficult parts are pushing up with their strength to a sitting or kneeling position.

Workers should ensure that the individual is not injured and does not wish to remain on the floor. When an injury occurs, the medical emergency must stabilise them and involve them in moving activity. Once it is confirmed that they are not injured, conscious and understand the moving activity, they can work with the care worker to be manually lifted off the floor.

One way to do this is for care workers to get them to sit on the floor with two workers kneeling on both sides of the service user and getting the service user to kneel with their hands using the chair on the floor.

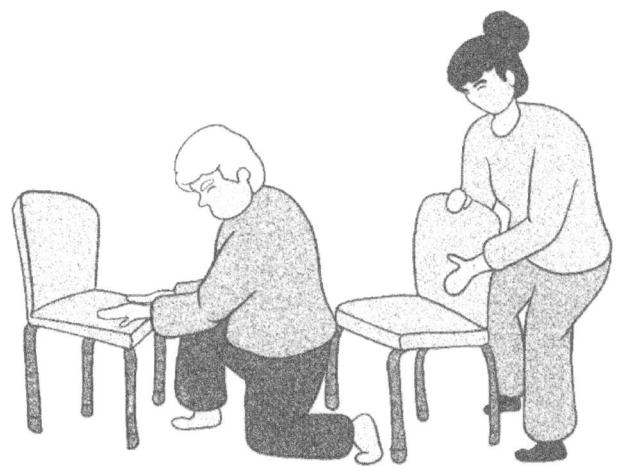

The service user uses the back of the chair to lift themselves into one knee from both knees, and the handling workers can support them in lifting off the floor with the other leg. This method may also require two pieces of sturdy furniture of different heights: a low stool, a bedside table, and an armchair. These are placed as close to the service user as possible.
(These methods are used when emergency service is not required).

Hoisting off the floor

The service user should be comfortable with a blanket or pillow while a lifting strategy is devised. This may require three or four handling workers to provide the service user with physical, emotional, and equipment support.

The process is as in a floor bed, by lowering the hoist. In addition to the hoisting procedure in the relevant section below, the following should be done:

- The hoist can be positioned at the head or foot end of a service user

Moving & Handling of People in Care Settings

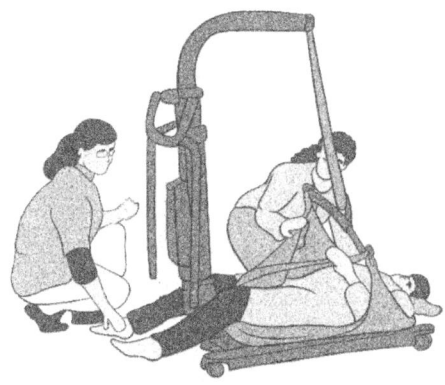

- Roll the service user onto the sling.
- Put a pillow under the head for comfort.
- Move the hoist closer, taking care of the spreader bar.
- Connect the slings with a short loop on the shoulders if to sit or a long loop if to put to bed.
- When using a hoist, keep the brakes off, follow the hoist and sling guide and avoid pushing over a long distance.

Controlling a Fall

If a worker thinks the service user is about to fall over, their fall can only be controlled to minimise the risk of injury. Supporting them is to prevent a full-impact fall without potentially injuring the worker.

In fall scenario:
1. Do not catch the person.
2. Do not pull the person over.
3. Control the fall by getting behind the service user, bending the knee and moving backwards as the

service user is lowered to the floor.
4. The worker may redirect their fall to avoid severe injury to the head.

Bariatric care

Another moving and handling challenge involves individuals above 159kgs or 25 stones. Their care and handling plan should classify them as bariatric. A Body Mass Index (BMI) table would have been used in risk assessment, and appropriate equipment would have been procured. Special training and equipment are also required to support such service users.

<u>Personal care</u>
According to the CQC, personal care supports people with activities like washing, bathing, toileting, cleaning themselves, getting dressed or going to the toilet for those who cannot care for these needs because of old age, illness, or disability. Personal care is a regulated activity that a barred worker cannot do. Care workers must be vetted through DBS to carry out this activity.

For personal reasons, service users may prefer a care worker of the same gender to assist them with personal care. Care workers of the opposite sex should not insert themselves into personal care activities where the service user has not made such requests and permission given.

Personal care requires support with the service user's mobility, even if temporary, and it is more likely that the same care workers providing personal care will be responsible for the moving and handling of the individual where equipment is required.

Personal care given by care workers should not involve nail cutting or grooming. Requests or needs for these should be made to the organisation to contact specialists for these services.

Special personal care training should be provided in line with full risk assessment and the care plan.

Unsafe / Controversial Lifting Techniques

Some lifting techniques are not deemed safe after being held controversial in the 80s and early 90s; however, it is difficult to say some are illegal as they have been known to be used in emergencies such as fire evacuation.
These unsafe techniques are:

Bed Drag Lift ✗
A lift off the bed that involves supporting an individual under the armpit using the worker's elbow crook. This technique puts pressure on the service user's shoulder and strains the lumbar region of the handling worker. The technique may also create shear force damage or bruises to the skin.

Chair Drag Lift ✗
It adopts the same technique as the bed drag lift but off the chair. In addition, this discourages the service user from being active in moving activities.

Standing Drag Lift ✗

Moving & Handling of People in Care Settings

As in the bed and chair drag lifts, this is also a controversial technique, with potential damage to the workers' elbows and an added risk of the service user falling over if they are disorientated by not seeing the direction of movement.

Bear Hug (Front & Back)

This technique resembles the pivot if engaged from the front. It involves leaning forward, marginal squatting and reaching forward around and under the arms of the individual and lifting them up and out of a surface. Unlike the pivot, however, it involves lifting over a longer distance.

It is unsafe for the worker as the full weight of the service user may now put an enormous strain on them. For the service user,

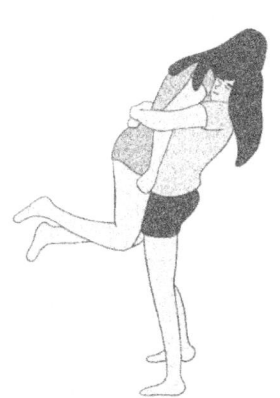
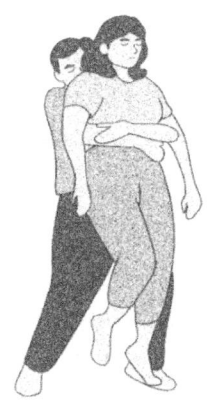

it may put pressure on their abdomen or breathing with the potential of falling over along with the worker.

Shoulder / Australian Lift

Moving & Handling of People in Care Settings

This unsafe technique involves two workers supporting the service user sitting up in bed. It anticipates a balance of the

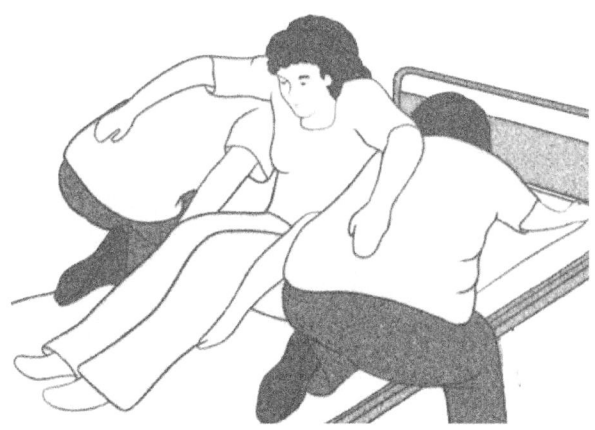

service user's weight between the workers. As this is always difficult, if not impossible, to achieve, the weight may tilt more heavily on one worker, especially if both workers are not of equal size in height and weight. This technique was commonly used for heavier individuals, possibly in the bariatric category.

Pivot Lift X

In transferring a service user from one surface, the pivot lift technique involves the service user standing up or squatting and "pivoting" on one or both feet with the workers supporting their weight and guiding them to spin to move their bottom to another surface.

The technique controversially involves linking arms behind the individual's back and pressuring their knees or thighs as they are

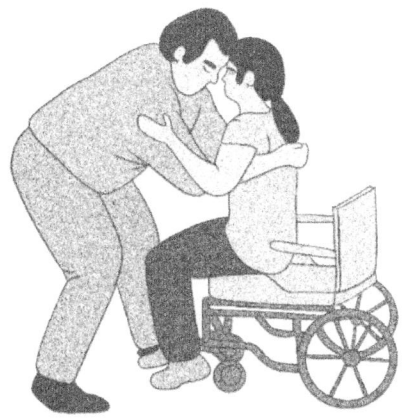

lifted. Some erroneously see this as safer than the drag lift, yet it is controversial because of the risk to the worker's back or falling with the service user if the latter has a weak lower body.

Through Arm Lift

This technique lifts a person from a surface with arms linked at

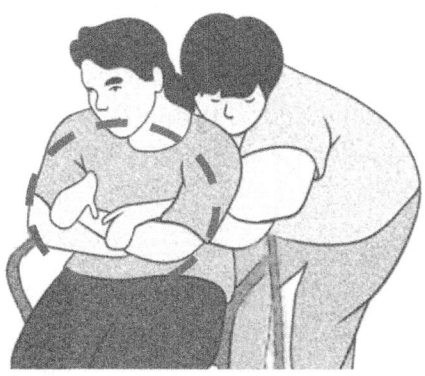

the front through the service user's armpits. This lift is operated at a distance from the worker's spine, putting strain on the spine, and there is a risk of twisting injury to the worker's shoulders and arms.

Blanket Lift (4)

This is not to be used in an emergency or life-threatening

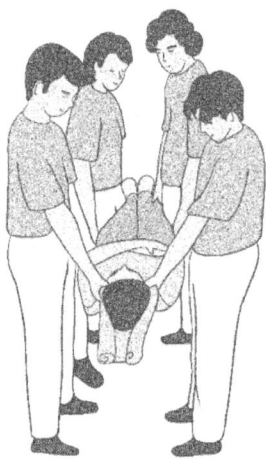

situation. It is designed to assist in transferring a sick or injured person out of extreme weather conditions.

Blanket Lift (6)

This technique is safe only when at least six workers or bystanders are available, plus a firm blanket long enough to support the individual's entire body.

Cradle Lift / Orthodox (Chair)

This controversial technique involves two workers standing on either side of the service user and forming a cradle with their hands, arms, and wrists to lift and move the individual. There is an immediate risk to the workers' lumbar region as the lift is done at arm's length. There are also risks to the individual under the knee or thigh.

Cradle Lift / Orthodox (Bed)

This is the same discredited and unsafe technique adopting the same principle as in chair lifting; however, lifting the service user from or to the bed poses a particular danger to the workers when used with a floor bed.

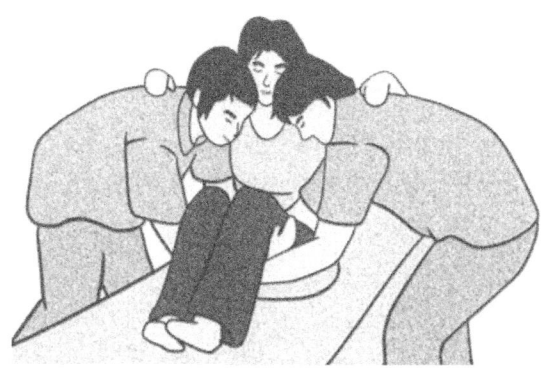

Hammock Lift

This arm and leg lift technique poses grave danger to the service user's spine and leg joints. It is a combination of through-arm lifts adopted by one worker whilst the other worker lifts the stretched legs of the individual.

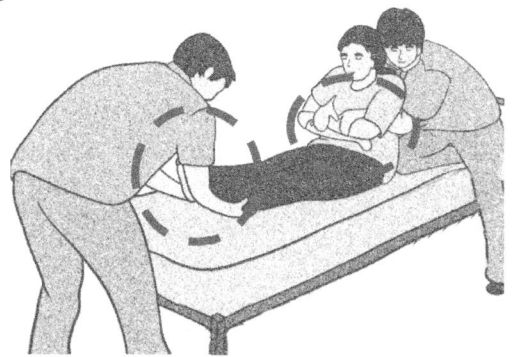

Other lifting safety guidelines
Where the individual is injured, the worker should:
1. Identify the injury type.
2. Get help.
3. Not move a person with a back injury unless they are in further immediate danger, such as a house fire threat.
4. Reassure the individual by telling them about the moving plan.
5. Employ the proper techniques.
6. Protect their back always.
7. Use the equipment on which workers have been trained to use.

Support & Comfort Aids

The type of equipment required for handling support will vary according to service users' specific needs. There are several aids and equipment, but not all are safe. Indeed, technology keeps increasing to make these aids safer than before. An example is the handling belt banned by the HSE for not lifting individuals but not for assisting individuals who can support their weight, such as in standing up.[45] The HSE has listed major ones, but this list is not exhaustive.[46]

Safety checks should be conducted before using all aids and equipment whilst workers read and follow the handling/hoisting plan. Care managers are encouraged to do an 'on-the-spot' risk assessment to ensure aids are not defective.

---

[45] https://www.hse.gov.uk/healthservices/moving-handling-equipment.htm
[46] *Ibid.*

Moving & Handling of People in Care Settings

List

- Adjustable Shower Chair
- Adjustable Trolley
- Bath Board
- Bath Lift
- Bath Mats
- Bath Seat
- Bath Step
- Bed Back Rest
- Bed Protectors
- Electric Bed
- Elephant Feet
- Fireside Chair
- Foot Stool
- Grab Bar
- Grab Rail
- Hand Reacher
- High Back Chair
- Hoist – Bed
- Hoist – Ceiling
- Hoist - Mobile
- Hoist – Standard
- Hoist – Standing
- Key safe
- Lifting cushions
- Mattress
- Multi Pill Dispenser
- Nursing Care Bed
- Overbed Table
- Perching Stool
- Pill Box
- Quad Recliner Bath Lift
- Riser Recliner Chair
- Raised Toilet Seat
- Ramp
- Rollator
- Rotating Seat
- Rotunda
- Bed table
- Belt - Transfer
- Can Opener
- Cane
- Care Bed
- Chair
- Chair table
- Commode
- Drinking System
- Seat
- Seat Cushion
- Sling - toileting
- Shower Stool with Rotating Sliding sheet – flat
- Sliding sheet – tubular
- Slings – Universal
- Sling - high
- Sling – amputee
- SOS Button
- Stair lifts
- Shoe Horn
- Shower Chair
- Shower Mats
- Shower Stool
- Stacking Commode
- Toilet Aid
- Toilet Frame
- Turn disc
- Triwalker
- Urinal – (male/female)
- Transfer Aid
- Transfer Aid – Seat to Stand
- Turntables
- Walking Frame
- Walking Stick
- Wheelchair

Selected aids/equipment and safe practices

Aids and equipment and their adaptation require the involvement of occupational therapists. Aids should be procured with a safety warranty, full manufacturer's instructions and PUWER/LOLER inspection certificate. They should also be aware of what care workers are trained in.

Seating: seats, including chairs, must fit the purpose. They should be safe and provide comfort. Some are adapted to meet service users' needs; however, general ergonomic seat design is essential for handling and use.

Before sitting, the service user must feel the back of the legs with the seat and sit slowly and gently, putting both hands on the seat handle if able. They may be guided on shuffling forward, backwards, or sideways to assist in moving.

Walking Frame: how the service user uses this device is up to them. The walking frame should be within their reach, be used unaided, and be unsuitable for those unable to walk. A frame is not to be used to support standing up. The height of the frame should be adjusted or ordered to suit the arm at an angle of 90 degrees.

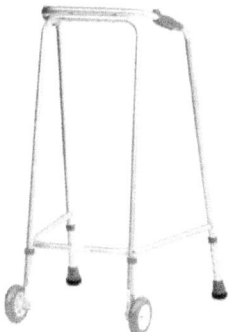

Moving & Handling of People in Care Settings

Walking Stick: like the walking frame, this also cannot be used as support for standing up and adjusted or ordered to suit the arm at an angle of 90 degrees.

Crutch: unlike a walking stick, the crutch offers more vital support and may be used in pairs.

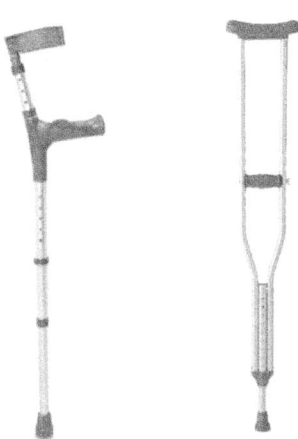

Handling belt: the HSE highlights the safe use of this aid. Handling belts should be held for use through loops at the Service user's back, getting them to push up on the arm of the chair. This device can aid in single-handed assistance to assist off a wheelchair.

Wheelchair

A wheelchair defines an individual's physical independence more than any other moving and handling aid. It may be manual or automatic, such as a rider-propelled type. Support is likely required for a service user in a manual wheelchair. Some devices also double up as a commode.

Requesting a ramp around the service user's home may be necessary for a wheelchair user. When using wheelchairs outdoors, workers should avoid shortcuts and follow a safe route.

Follow the wheelchair usage guidelines for safety:
For example:
- Avoid lifting the wheelchair with a person in it
- Ensure they have their feet on the footplates before transportation
- Use a seatbelt
- Always put on the brakes when the wheelchair is stationary
- Check brakes and tyre pressure regularly
- Avoid using over kerbs

Moving a person from a wheelchair into a car:
- Open the car door wide
- Remove the side of the wheelchair nearest to the car
- Position the wheelchair as close to the car as possible, at a slight angle
- Put the wheelchair brakes on
- Using the same technique as helping someone out of a chair
- Protect the individual's head from hitting the top of the door frame when lowered into the car

Bed/mattress
A bed could be a standard profile or floor bed. The latter is appropriate for those who fall off a standard profile bed and risk injuring themselves.

Bed rails may be added for safety. Care workers should lower the bed to work if a rail is present. They should also lower the bed if hoisting, as it is better and safer to lower the bed than raise the hoist.

Electric profiling beds (EPBs) have proven to reduce the risks of injuries in workers while providing greater comfort and independence for service users. These beds make it easier for service users to sit up in bed. It also aids in easier bracket and height adjustments, reducing workers' stooping or overreaching. EPBs are generally heavier than standard non-profiling beds, increasing the risks from moving them, and there are risks of damage to electric or trailing cables that can cause electrocution or a trip hazard.

The worker should pay attention to mattress designs as they may indicate the direction of the head or feet. Mattresses usually have special coverings for hygiene purposes.

Attention should also be paid to bedding, such as mattress covers, sheets, blankets, duvets, or quilts, and how the service user wants it laid.

Bed table

There are various bed-table types, and they should have adjustable heights. A tilting table can be used flat for eating, drinking or book reading, and some are sturdy enough to be rested on when tilted.

Commode

This may be built into a wheelchair or fixed chair. A commode is an essential personal care device. A hygiene procedure must be strictly followed when handling a commode.

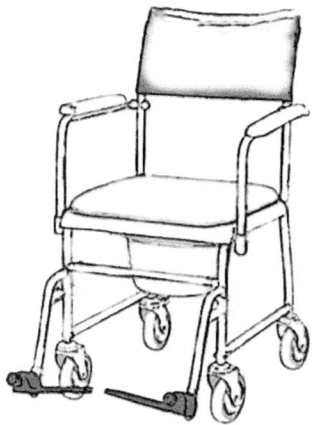

Sliding sheets
These are in sheets or tubular form, enabling the service user to move without causing friction from dragging or pulling.
They can be used:
- To move individuals up the bed
- Get their legs out of bed
- Make transfer boards more effective
- Relieve service users with pressure sores (ulcers) during turning or hoisting because they reduce friction on bottoms, shoulders, or heels

Lying to sitting using sliding sheets
This activity requires two workers:
- While on the bed, insert sliding sheets beneath the service user as they are turned to the side
- The second worker pulls the sliding sheets, and the service user is turned to the other side
- When the sliding sheets are in place, turn the service user slowing at an angle of 90 degrees with one worker always supporting their head
- The service user is supported to sit up while one worker

gently pulls the sliding sheet to swivel the bed's edge in the direction the service user wishes to sit
- A turn-disc can be used while inserted under the buttocks, and a slide sheet under the legs to swivel around on the bed to sit over the edge of the bed

Transfer board

Also known as a sliding board, this is a flat and rigid board made of wood or plastic. It could be straight, curved or boomerang in shape. A transfer board is designed to support physical disability by moving from one surface, like a bed, to another surface, such as a chair, commode, or wheelchair. It can be used along with a sliding sheet even for better outcomes.

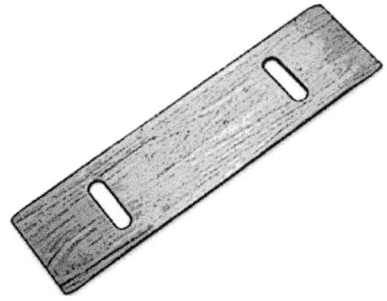

A board is primarily used in an assisted transfer activity but can also be used independently by service users. Service users need reasonable upper body control to use a sliding board.

Sling

A sling is a supporting belt or harness used with a hoist or standing aid to move a service user safely from one point to another. It is used for limited mobility, particularly personal care, toileting or transfers. By regulation, a sling must be LOLER compliant by being assessed, regularly checked, fit for purpose, and compatible with the hoist.

Slings vary in size, with some having neck and head support and must be for the hoist identified. It must not be used if this label is faded or damaged. The manufacturer's label on the slings provides safety information on usage.

During use, workers must double-check that the loops/clips are properly attached to the spreader bar throughout the activity.

A sling must not be removed from a service user's workplace or exchanged for another service user. This may differ in a care home where one sling may fit more than one service user. However, there should be a hygiene procedure for mixed-use. The toileting sling should not be used for several service users in a care home.

The habit of leaving a sling on the hoist after use is incorrect; it should be folded away after use.

For male users, ensure that the bottom double straps do not hurt them in between the thighs.

Toileting and its pitfalls
Safer equipment for toileting is a standing hoist; however, a transfer from chair to commode will be possible for a service user with good upper body strength after they have been undressed (in the chair) and are ready for toileting. Using a sliding sheet on the sliding board will reduce friction for this activity.

Hoisting

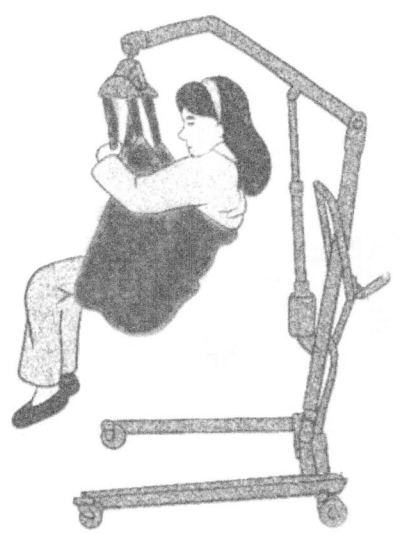

Hoisting legislation
Hoisting is a regulated activity highlighted by several legislations; however, LOLER Regulation 5 requires suitable slings to support mobile or fixed hoists to handle individuals. More information on hoist-safe use is in HSE's *Getting to Grips with Hoisting People*.

HSE and MHRA are concerned about the increasing number of serious injury reports yearly. Injuries commonly associated with poor hoisting and where hoisting guidelines are ignored are:

- Bruises
- Broken bones
- Skin lacerations
- Death

An average of 120 incidents per year regarding hoisting accidents are reported to the MHRA. These are related to the following:
- Wrong sling size
- Wrong hoist type
- Hoist instability
- Single-handed care instead of two-handed

Hoisting legislation also covers training and sling.

Training
An operator of the hoist should have received up-to-date training.

Appropriate Sling
Handlers/operators must ensure the appropriate sling is clean and compatible with the named service user and the hoist.

Hoisting risk assessment
According to HSE, however, hosting guidelines should start with risk assessment under the MHOR with recourse to the care plan and an up-to-date handling/hoisting plan.

The hoisting risk assessment should consider the TILEO acronym of the **t**ask, **i**ndividual, **l**oad (person) and **e**nvironment, adding "**o**" for **o**ther factors, such as equipment.

Most hoists require a double-handed approach/rota of care workers. However, it should not be surprising that local authorities are promoting aids and equipment with advanced technology that try to turn some double-handed moving and handling activities into single-handed ones to reduce costs.

Hoisting Environment[47]
Workers must ensure that:
- the environment is ready for the task;
- there is ample space around all around for safe hoisting;
- the floor is clear of obstacles;
- there is a safe area for storing and charging the hoist.

Hoisting checklist and additional guidance according to Legislation [48]

Checks handling workers must carry out before use:
See the Initial and Equipment Checks Guidelines tables below and in addition:
- Are handlers trained?
- Have handlers read and followed a current and relevant handling/hoisting plan?
- Is it decided that this is a single or double-handed activity?
- Are more workers required?
- Is the environment safe and appropriate, and is space sufficient and clear of danger with floor level and free of obstacles?
- Is the hoisting destination ready and safe to receive the service user?
- Are attachments secured and the individual safe before proceeding?

Checks handling workers must carry out during the tasks:
See During the Tasks Guidelines table below and in addition:
- When connecting the sling to the hoist, the spreader bar/carry bar should be brought down slowly with attention to avoiding contact injuries with the individual.

---

[47] HSE (20110 "Getting to grips with hoisting people". Health Service Information Sheet 3
[48] *Ibid.*

- Communicate with everyone always involved in the task.
- Reassure the individual at all times and involve them as much as possible.
- Ensure the safety and comfort of the individual always.
- If there are concerns about the equipment, task, individual, environment, etc., handlers must follow organisational procedures immediately.
- Hoist the individual just above the surface from which they are being lifted to obtain sufficient clearance.
- Do not leave the individual unattended in a hoist.
- The individual must consistently and reliably bear weight through their legs and have sufficient upper-body muscle strength/sitting balance.
- The individual must be able to cooperate and physically participate in the hoisting process.

Checks handling workers must carry out after the tasks:
See After the Tasks Guidelines table below and in addition:
- Store the hoist in a safe place with the spreader bar in the lowest position and brakes on when unused.

Additional checks specific to Standard and Mobile Hoists
1. Ensure the hoist is not connected to electricity.
2. The hoist brakes should be off during hoisting to avoid tilting, as hoists are designed to self-balance.
   Note: There are certain types of equipment where the brakes need to be applied, which will be highlighted.
3. The hoist base legs should be open.
4. The lower the hoist, the more stable it is.
5. Service users must face the direction of the hoist travel, not inward.
6. Apply the sling on the service user first and bring the hoist in last.

Moving & Handling of People in Care Settings

7. Avoid using the hoist to transport over long distances and thresholds unless stated in the handling plan.

Additional checks specific to Track / Overhead / Ceiling Hoist[49]
1. The hoist motor should be directly overhead, and the lifting tape should be vertical to the lift. This will avoid malfunctioning and reduce wear and tear.
2. The hoist tracking must always be clear of obstructions.
3. When not used, the spreader bar should be elevated to its highest position and returned to its docking station.

Additional checks specific to Bath Hoists[50]
1. Special attention must be paid to the environment regarding a slippery/wet floor, bath, and shower, as bath oils, bubble baths, lotion, etc., may increase the risks of accidents.
2. Test the water temperature.

Hoisting off the floor *(see above)*

Hoisting to/off the bed

1. Two workers will be required unless the hoist is fully electric and the service user with the required capacity can actively participate in the difficult tasks.
2. Depending on the original position, such as a chair or wheelchair, the service user's femur must be comfortable and ready for bed to assist in positioning the service user.
3. When using a hoist, keep brakes off, follow the sling guide if provided, and take care of posture whilst

---

[49] ibid
[50] ibid

Moving & Handling of People in Care Settings

    manoeuvring the hoist, and avoid pushing over long distances.
4. As a basic rule, workers should regularly check the comfort and safety of service users.

<u>Hoisting guidelines</u>
Hoisting, generally, is safe and dignified. Several organisations, such as the NBE, have developed guidelines with HSE to ensure safe hoisting practices in all service areas.

Health and social care service providers have benefited from this HSE collaboration with other organisations. However, they should develop policies and procedures through these within the context of caregiving and the content of their workers' training programmes.

Organisations can adapt the tables below for use. They indicate significant steps and checks in hoisting operation reflecting the following sections:

1. Initial Checks
2. Equipment checks before operation.
3. Checks during the activity,
4. Checks after the activity.

GUIDELINES FOR USING HOISTS & SLINGS
Initial Checks

Before the Task: Initial Checks

- Have you had up-to-date moving & handling training, including hoisting training?
  - No → DO NOT USE / Check with supervisor
  - Yes ↓
- Do you feel confident using the hoist?
  - No → Check with supervisor
  - Yes ↓
- Is there a current and person-specific care / handling plan for the hoist?
  - No → Check with supervisor
  - Yes ↓
- Is the person's condition the same as when they were assessed for this particular equipment?
  - No → Check with supervisor
  - Yes ↓
- Do you have the person's consent?
  - No → Check with supervisor
  - Yes ↓
- Does the number of care workers assigned for this task tally with what is assessed in the care plan?
  - No → Check with supervisor
  - Yes ↓
- Are you familiar with this specific hoist / sling?
  - No → Check with supervisor
  - Yes ↓
- Is the area safe for hoisting?
  Is there sufficient space?
  Is it clear of obstacles?
  Is it clean and dry?
  Is there access around / under the furniture?
  - No → Check with supervisor / DO NOT USE
  - Yes

GUIDELINES FOR USING HOISTS & SLINGS
Equipment Checks

Before the Task: Equipment Checks

If the environment is safe for hoisting:

- Are you familiar with the hoist's emergency stop? — **No** → DO NOT USE Check with supervisor / **Yes** ↓

- Is the sling compatible for use with this hoist? — **No** → DO NOT USE / **Yes** ↓

- Is sling the one identified in the care / handling plan and still appropriate in terms of type and size? — **No** → DO NOT USE / **Yes** ↓

- Have you made visual checks of the sling? Is it clean, undamaged? Are labels legible and with unique identifier? Is LOLER examination up to date (6 monthly)? — **No** → DO NOT USE / **Yes** ↓

- Have you made visual checks of the hoist? Is the battery charged? Are there signs of damage? Does the hoist move freely on castors forwards and backwards? Are the lifting / lowering mechanism moving freely? Is the emergency button set in correct position? Is LOLER examination up to date (6 monthly)? — **No** → DO NOT USE Check with supervisor / **Yes** ↓

Commence hoisting task

GUIDELINES FOR USING HOISTS & SLINGS
During the Task

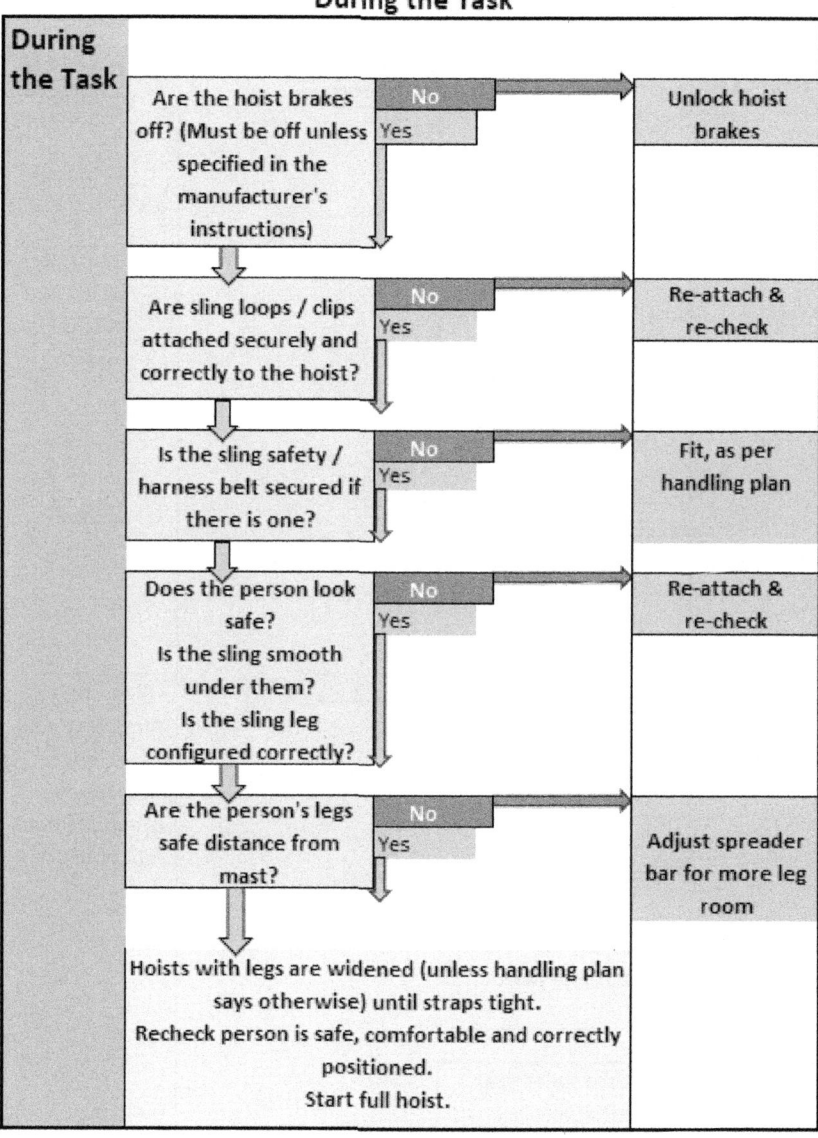

Moving & Handling of People in Care Settings

GUIDELINES FOR USING HOISTS & SLINGS
After the Task

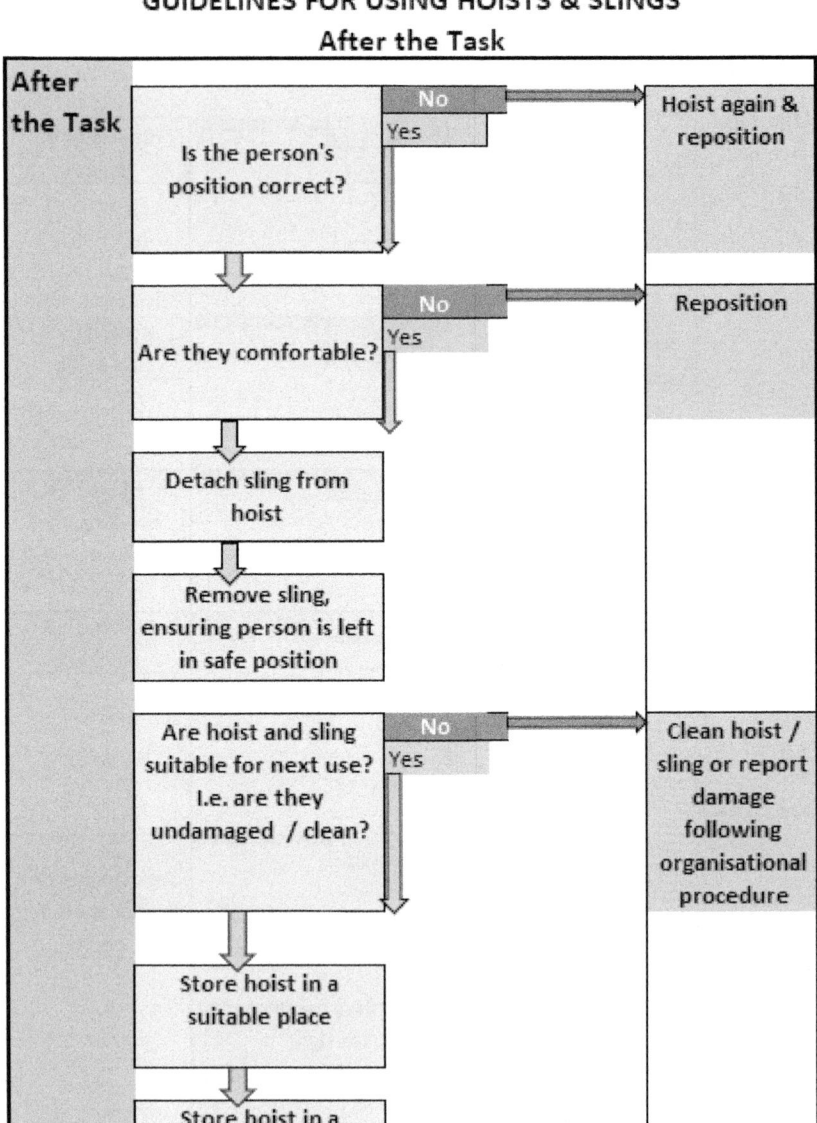

Chapter Seven
Training & Professional Development

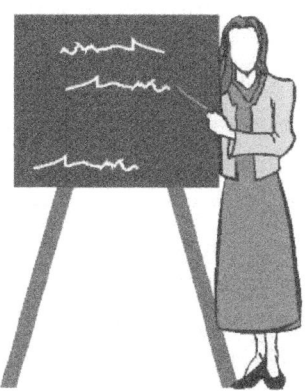

Knowledge, Understanding and Skills in Manual Handling of Objects

<u>Importance of skills acquisition in manual handling</u>
Knowledge is a sum of what is known about a subject acquired through experience or education, while understanding enables reflection and appraisal of the subject. Skill is the ability to do something well, attaining expertise in a task.

Knowledge and understanding do not keep people safe, but their applications in skills do. Improved skills reduce abuse, neglect, harm or exploit in moving and handling, enabling the care workers to do things better and smarter. It is a required skill to put into action the knowledge and understanding of the legislation to ensure workers act within the law.

Besides knowledge and understanding, skill is another attribute of achieving the goal of moving and handling objects and People. Knowledge and understanding gained at induction or initial training can only improve well-being when further skills and experience are acquired in refresher training.

Skills are more important in moving and handling people than inanimate objects. This is because a holistic approach is more relevant in the case of people over and above the knowledge and understanding of manual handling techniques and equipment handling, as can be seen in the case of the relevance of the skills in communication, respect, nutrition, etc.

Skill ensures that the worker attains competence quickly and thoroughly to follow correct procedures for the service user and preserve their dignity. There should also be a skill in seeking the service user's consent to agree and accept the moving activities and processes.

Finally, skill is required to ensure the correct equipment use, management and update on advances in the technology embedded in the equipment.

Three principles of achieving and applying skills are:
- Stop
- Think
- Assess

Research
Since MHOR 27 confirms that research in manual handling has found little evidence that handling techniques-focused training is effective in promoting a safer working environment and reducing injuries, training professional development approaches should, therefore, change and be holistic-focused.

What is also apparent is that handling techniques-focused

Moving & Handling of People in Care Settings

training may reduce injuries, as a matter of legislation concern, in activities linked to the equipment. It is only through a holistic foundation that non-technique-based injuries can be reduced.

MHOR confirms that some research shows strong evidence that injuries can be reduced by multi-dimensional ergonomics interventions involving workers, managers, equipment and/or task redesign, and person-centred training. Such findings emphasise:
- change in attitudes and behaviour
- promoting risk awareness
- reporting concerns

Therefore, it seems that a holistic approach, compliance with equipment use guidelines and RIDDOR will improve the working environment while reducing injuries.

The organisational management
The management should oversee training within the organisation. It should ensure staff involvement at all levels, particularly supervisors and managers responsible for risk assessment. Managers should also update themselves with a holistic understanding of care in order to adequately mentor workers.

There should be posters or display notices on injuries and potential risks to workers in moving and handling. A safe training environment with a good supervision culture and effective timetable should provide trainers with responsibility for as few trainees as possible.

Formal training, particularly induction and onsite training supervision, should follow with similar equipment used for training.

The Trainer

A trainer in moving and handling people should be qualified and versatile in health and social care knowledge. They should know about industry compliance and technical knowledge of aids in moving and handling, as well as common equipment for care work.

Likewise, a trainer's knowledge of service users' needs and safety concerns in general, the care workers' (trainees) attitudes and work ethics, and the organisation's approaches are paramount and should be ahead of training techniques where such techniques will not directly impact the work environment positively.

It is a health and safety at work requirement for employers to provide training on crucial health and safety risks. Guidance in MHOR covers specific moving and handling activities to complement this requirement. This is because a healthcare workplace setting poses significant moving and handling challenges and risks.

Trainers should refresh their moving and handling PDP every three years at least to keep up to date and, in the interim, attend manual handling programmes or workshop opportunities offered by local authorities.

Both in-house and external trainers should ensure that the training equipment they display or work with complies with regulations, particularly PUWER and LOLER.

Mandatory Training

Training programmes designed for induction and refresher sessions should be mandatory, with modules reflecting the organisation's needs.

Induction training should follow the Care Certificate standards (or similar) adapted for moving and handling and personal care. Indeed, trainers should ensure that organisations are not encouraged to send workers into the field without induction training and pass training assessments on personal care, moving and handling techniques, medication administration and policies and procedures of their employing organisations. A moving and handling induction training should last at least one or two days, and the practical aspect should not be online. Shadowing should follow immediately after induction training.

Some employers risk sending new staff to "shadow" before training. This will only steer such workers toward the wrong attitudes and work ethics in the future.

A refresher training should be interactive and focus on filling gaps in skills. Workers should be able to share experiences guided by the trainer to protect service users' confidentiality. Refresher learners should demonstrate robust pre-assessments, where health and social care knowledge and skills can be evidenced. The HSE and the CSA2002 recommend that the employer set frequent refresher training and the required training for a new role before commencing tasks and duties.

All moving and handling training sessions should be certified and count towards the count learner's CPD. Learners should learn to create their PDP to help focus on specific areas of development which the organisation should either sponsor, subsidise or support. The national minimum requirement should apply where there is proficiency in literacy, internet, numeracy, and communication skills. Learners should evidence these core and reporting skills.

Training should be supported by workplace supervisors with practical instructions and competence assessments on using any mechanical aids provided for undertaking moving and handling tasks. If a staff member or learner does not meet the required level of current knowledge, understanding, and practice through pre-assessment, they should complete the induction again.

Legislation and Strategies for Training in Moving and Handling

Legislation on manual handling training
The provisions of MHOR, MHSWR, RIDDOR and the CA2014 are apparent in the requirement for training compliance by organisations, care workers and other parties involved in the care of moving and handling.

The following areas are covered or implied in the above legislation:
- Duty of care
- Holistic approach to care
- Risk Assessments
- Risk factors and how injuries can happen
- Appropriate work systems for the individual's tasks and environment
- Use of mechanical aids
- Safe manual handling and good handling techniques
- Reporting symptoms and injuries

- Responsibilities of trainers
- Practical work relevant to the job allows trainers to highlight and correct what trainees are not doing correctly
- Responsibilities of organisations for training compliance
- Responsibilities of care workers to subject themselves to training
- Records and evidence of training
- Training updates, refreshers and CPD
- The information covered by manual handling training should be specific to the job

A trainer will guide learners to comply with the law and follow best practices by ensuring these topics are training content.

Suggested Holistic Lesson Plan

In training, the following checklist of the Lesson plan can be adapted:
1. Introduction and Housekeeping.
2. Provide Training Agreement (see *below*).
3. Create Individual Training Records (see *below*).
4. Learning Outcomes.
5. Training Structure:
   PART 1
   a. Importance of well-being
   b. Legislation
   c. Structure of the human back and injuries
   d. Service user's physical and mental capacities
   e. Risk Assessments
   f. Incidents, accidents and injuries
   g. Loads, people and non-people
   h. Nutrition and well-being
   i. Dignity and self-care

   j. Communication, confidentiality and reporting
 PART 2
   k. Health and safety, COSHH and infections
   l. Local issues, policies and procedures
   m. Safe and unsafe activities
   n. Ergonomics approach and technological aids
   o. Practical session
6. Training Assessment –
   Tests and answers during the session
   Individual Learning Record – indicating techniques, if discussed, demonstrated, practised, and achieved.

Training tips

1. Housekeeping sessions should include trainees' welfare conveniences, health and safety checks, respect for others in class and decorum.
2. The inclusion and diversity policy is to be included in the housekeeping session.
3. Learning Outcomes are to be stated clearly and checked in summary.
4. Provide enough comfort breaks for refreshments.
5. Handouts/handbooks should be provided.
6. Workbooks should be provided and marked.
7. There should be sufficient time to acquire the necessary skills.
8. Training should be geared towards the learners' competency.
9. Training must focus on all equipment that is to be used in the workplace.
10. General well-being factors, such as nutrition, communication, etc., should be identified.
11. Refreshers should focus on the following:

a. Updating skills following assessment of the individual's competence.
   b. Outcomes of any local audits.
   c. Monitoring reports of their performance and considering changes to their tasks.
   d. Equipment or new developments in moving and handling policy and practice.
   e. Local Authority requirement.
   f. Safeguarding.
12. Feedback should be incorporated into the training programme. In class exercises, feedback amongst learners should be included.
13. Moving and handling training should not be conducted wholly online. The practical part should be face-to-face, at least.

Examples of practical demonstration and assessment

1. Positioning of the individual
2. Sit to Stand (minimal assistance)
3. Stand to Sit (facing towards)
4. Assisted shuffle / rock forward in a chair
5. Assisted walking
6. Safety of walking frame
7. Transfer from chair to wheelchair, and vice versa
8. Using a stand-and-turn transfer aid
9. Using a Turntable for a weaker leg
10. Crouch transfer using a turntable
11. Assisting into and out of bed
12. Lying to sitting
13. Using a slide sheet
14. Using transfer boards
15. Falling individual
16. Climbing up/down the stairs

17. Emergency handling
18. Working in confined spaces
19. Personal care, if agreed
20. Other demonstrations that the organisation may identify

Other Matters for Consideration

Recommended further training after induction
1. Children
2. Disability
3. Refresher for trainers
4. First Aid
5. Dealing with pressure/bed sores

Factors that may impact moving and handling in the future
1. Artificial intelligence
2. Development in aids and equipment technology
3. Lack of funding
4. Privatisation of care
5. Care workers' contracts

Employing organisation

1. The organisation should have a training audit to check that individual employees follow regulations, policies, and procedures.
2. They should ensure that learning facilitators are physically capable of demonstrating good practice in all aspects of moving and handling and having the appropriate qualifications, experience, or background to deliver training to a satisfactory standard. Such

facilitators should be DBS-checked to legally visit service users for inspections, observations, or assessments.
3. Organisations should provide a suitable permanent means of safe access to operate the equipment for storage, inspection, maintenance, and repair.

Training Records

<u>Individual learning record</u>
This document should evidence the following:
1. Organisation's name.
2. Date of activity training.
3. The activities involving hoist, sliding sheet, transfer board, wheelchair, double/single-handed techniques, etc.
4. Discussion feedback.
5. Demonstration feedback.
6. Assignment feedback.
7. Final assessment if achieved or not achieved.
8. Learner's name and signature.
9. Trainer / Assessor's name and signature.

<u>Training Agreement</u>
This document should evidence the following:
1. Organisation's name.
2. Date of moving and handling training.
3. Foreword highlighting – *trainees would be involved in individual and group practical activities, and advise them not to go beyond the instructions.*
4. Disclosure – *A short statement mandating the trainee to disclose any medical or physical reasons, including current or historic*

musculoskeletal problems, injuries or other health conditions such as pregnancy, why they cannot participate.
5. Warning – *A short statement warning trainees not to expose themselves or others to physical harm.*
6. Table – *is suggested for opportunities to list possible physical injuries or concerns that trainees may have.*
7. Confirmation – by the learner that they understand the Agreement.
8. Learner's name, signature and date.
9. Manager or Trainer or Assessor's name, signature and date.

Workbook
Completed by the trainee, assessed, signed and dated by the trainer/assessor with feedback.

Training certificate
This could be an Attendance Certificate or an Award by a regulated certification body that will include the following:
1. Training Organisation.
2. Trainee's name.
3. Employing organisation/sponsor.
4. Course title.
5. Learning outcome.
6. Training date.
7. Certificate issue date, if different.
8. Certificate expiry date.
9. Certificate's authorised signatory.
10. Certificate number.

Chapter Eight
Conclusion

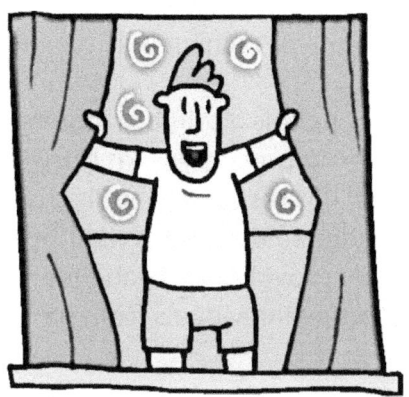

In summary

The holistic approach taken by this manual is necessary, timely, and informed. It is necessary because it takes up the often-ignored challenge of legislation MHOR 27, which asserts that research does not support the effectiveness of lifting techniques-focused manual handling training in promoting a safer working environment that various legislations set out to establish.

If, indeed, as evidence suggests, relying on the same legislation, techniques taught in training programmes often fail to be applied in the workplace, then a change in training approach is not only necessary but also overdue.

Not many resources have been produced since the devastating COVID-19 pandemic, which changed our way of working and learning, even in health and social care. People living in care settings suffered higher death rates, isolation, and sometimes cognitive and functional decline, and healthcare workers' health also suffered.[51] Working and learning remotely has not helped to improve actual care and well-being as care roles are still yet to be filled and face-to-face training fully resumed.

Wanting to do what is right is a primary requirement for a change in attitude. This is precisely what MHOR seeks to promote. This manual has responded to that challenge by providing the knowledge to do what is right by law and best practices. It has solidly provided ways and means of providing well-being and protecting individuals from harm during moving and handling activities.

Organisations are also reminded of their obligations to create and foster the necessary, safe environment through compliant policies, procedures, robust risk assessment culture and support for the proper training.

As a training guide, this manual boldly offers a different approach for care workers to inculcate the right attitude through awareness of their legal obligations to the individuals for whom they. Within this awareness, they can carry out the physical aspects of moving and handling with due care for the safety of those in the workplace, including themselves and their service users.

Awareness should consider the individual's well-being regarding nutrition, protection from infections, independence, and respectful communication, and focus on compliance with

---

[51] BMA, 2023 Report, pp15-17.

Moving & Handling of People in Care Settings

policies and procedures and avoiding safeguarding pitfalls. This holistic approach addresses the person-centred needs factors surrounding workers' attitudes, knowledge, understanding, and skill enhancement to work safely.

Kindly recommend this manual to others and leave a review on Amazon or at info@claritaspublishing.co.uk

Bibliography

Books & Journals
Carer's Handbook, 1997, *A Practical Guide to Looking after Ill, Disabled, and Elderly People,* Dorling Kindersley Book, London.
Carers UK, *State of Caring 2022: A snapshot of unpaid care in the UK*, November 2022.
Cherney, A. and Head, B., 2011, Evidence and Policy, 7(4), November 2011, *Supporting the knowledge-to-action process: a systems-thinking approach.* pp.471-488, Policy Press, Bristol.
Gershlick, B. and Charlesworth, A., 2019, "Health and social care workforce: Priorities for the next government". The Health Foundation, England.
Moudatsou, Maria, et al., 2020, The Role of Empathy in *Health and Social Care Professionals*, MDPI, Basel.
Peace, D. and Atkinson, R., 2019, *Holistic approaches to safeguarding adolescents,* University of Bedfordshire. Contextual Safeguarding Network, Bedford.
Ruszala, S. et al., 2010, *Standards in Manual Handling,* (3rd edition), National Back Exchange, Towcester.
Shapiro, J., 2002, "How do physicians teach empathy in the primary care setting", *Acad. Med.* 2002, 77, 323–329, CrossRef, PubMed.
Smith, J., (ed.), 2011, *The Guide to the Handling of People, A Systems Approach,* 6th edition, Backcare, Teddington.
Sturman-Floyd, M., 2013, "Moving and handling: assessing the handler", *Nursing and Residential Care,* 15(2), 2013, pp.98-101, MA Healthcare Ltd., London.
Wells, J., 1998, *The Home Care Workers Handbook, The Essential Guide to Care in the Home,* UKHCA Ltd, Surrey.

Documents
Back in work – Back Pack 22 June 2010 found at ww.nhsemployers.org/HealthyWorkplaces/MSDs/Pages/Backinwork-backpack.aspx {accessed 1/11/2023}.
British Medical Association, 2023, *The impact of the pandemic on population health and health inequalities,* London.
Department of Health, *Self care – A real choice: Self care support – A practical option,* 2005.
Directorate for Health & Social Care Integration, 2014, *The Scottish Manual Handling Passport Scheme,* also found at https://www.hse.gov.uk/scotland/

pdf/manual-passport.pdf
European Framework Directive on Safety and Health at Work, 1989.
HSE, 2011, *Getting to grips with hoisting people* HSIS3.
HSE, 2014. *Health and Safety in Care Homes*. HSG22
HSE, 2012, *How the Lifting Operations and Lifting Equipment Regulations apply to health and social care,* Health Services Information Sheet 4 (rev1) HSIS4.
HSE, 2018, *Manual handling assessment charts (the MAC tool),* INDG383(rev3).
HSE, 2020, *Manual handling at work: A brief guide,* INDG143(rev4).
HSE, *Risk assessment: A brief guide to controlling risks in the workplace,* INDG163 (rev4), found at https://www.hse.gov.uk/simple-health-safety/risk/index.htm {accessed 3/1/2024}.
HSE, 2016, *Risk assessment of pushing and pulling (RAPP) tool,* INDG478.
HSE, 2002, *The Manual Handling Operations Regulations 1992,* (as Amended 2002).
HSE, 2014, *Safe use of lifting equipment. Lifting Operations and Lifting Equipment Regulations 1998.* Approved Code of Practice and Guidance, L113 (Second edition), Regulation 5.
HSE, 2013, *Consulting employees on health and safety: A brief guide to the law,* INDG232 (rev2).
HSE, 2023, *Health and safety statistics,* found at https://www.hse.gov.uk/statistic {accessed between 4/6/23 and 31/01/24}.
ISO Technical Report, 2012, TR 12296, "Ergonomics – Manual Handling of People in the Health Care Sector". Also found at http://www.iso.org/iso/home/store /catalogue_tc/catalogue_detail .htm?csnumber=51310 {accessed 31/09/2023}.
National Back Exchange, 2018, *Code of Professional Conduct.*
NHS Digital, 2022, "Adult Social Care Statistics in England: An Overview".
Skills for Care, *The Care Certificate.*
The Office of National Statistics 2022, also found at https://www.ons.gov.uk/peoplepopulationandcommunity/healthandsocialcare
The Office for National Statistics, 2024, Earnings and hours worked, care workers: ASHE Table 26 found at https://www.ons.gov.uk/search?q=care+worker {accessed 20/01/2024}.
The Office for Statistics Regulations, 2020, Adult Social Care Statistics in England. OSR, London.
Trainer Courses Limited, *Manual Handling Resource,* Version V1.4., 2020.

Moving & Handling of People in Care Settings

Relevant Legislation
Care Act of 2014
Control of Substances Hazardous to Health Regulations 2002
Equality Act 2010
General Data Protection Regulations 2018
Health and Safety at Work etc Act 1974
Health and Social Care Act 2008
Lifting Operations and Lifting Equipment Regulations 1998
Manual Handling Operations Regulations 1992
Management of Health and Safety at Work Regulations 1999
Mental Capacity Act 2005
Reporting of Injuries, Diseases and Dangerous Occurrences Regulations 2013
Provision and Use of Work Equipment Regulations 1998

Other online sources
https://en.wikipedia.org/wiki/Human_back
https://www.bma.org.uk/advice-and-support/covid-19/what-the-bma-is-doing/the-impact-of-the-pandemic-on-population-health-and-health-inequalities
https://www.gov.uk/government/publications/care-act-2014-part-1-factsheets/care-act-factsheets
http://www.hse.gov.uk/statistics/overall/hssh1617.pdf
http://www.hse.gov.uk/toolbox/manual.htm
http://www.hse.gov.uk/legislation/hswa.htm
http://www.hse.gov.uk/msd/pushpull/regulations.htm
http://www.hse.gov.uk/work-equipment-machinery/puwer.htm
http://www.hse.gov.uk/work-equipment-machinery/loler.
https://www.nhs.uk/conditions/slipped-disc/
https://rospaworkplacesafety.com/2013/02/18/manual-handling-definition/
http://www.hse.gov.uk/pubns/indg143.pdf
https://lead-academy.org/blog/illegal-moving-and-handling-techniques/
https://ledezmalawfirm.com/injuries/spine-injuries/
https://medical-dictionary.thefreedictionary.com/dorsum
https://www.safetybusiness.co.uk
https://www.spineinfo.com/anatomy/intervertebral-discs-structure-function-and-disorders/

Moving & Handling of People in Care Settings

Organisations that support better moving and handling of people

Alzheimer's Disease Society, Gordon House, 10 Green coat Place, London SW1P 1PH, *www.alzheimers.org.uk*
    Scotland: **Action on Dementia**, 22 Drumsbeugh Gardens Edinburgh EH3 7RN, *www.alzscot.org*

Arthritis Care, 18 Stephenson Way, London, NW1 2HD, *www.arthritiscare.org.uk*
Back Care, 16 Elm Tree Road, Teddington, Middlesbrough, TW11 8ST, *www.backwards.org.uk*
Black Disabled People's Group, c/o Greater London Association of Disabled People
336 Brixton Road, London, SW9 7AA, *www.glad.org.uk*
British Association of Occupational Therapists, 106-114 Borough High Street, London, SE1 1LB, *www.cot.org.uk*
Brittle Bone Society, 30 Guthrie Street, Dundee, DD1. 5BS, *www.brittlebone org*
Chartered Society of Physiotherapy, 14 Bedford Row, London, WC1R 4ED, *www.csp.org.uk*
Citizens Advice Bureau CAB, Myddleton House, 115-123 Pentonville Road London, *www.citizensadvice.org.uk*
Dementia UK, 7th Floor, One Aldgate, London EC3N 1RE, *www.dementiauk.org*
Department of Health, Richmond House, 79 Whitehall, London, SW1A 2NS, *www.doh.gov.uk*
Disabled Living Centres Council, 1st Floor, Winchester House, 11 Crammer Road
London SW9 6EJ, *www.disabledliving.co.uk*
General Social Care Council, Skipton House, London Road, London SE1 6LH, *www.scie.org.uk*
    Scotland: Scottish Social Services Council, Compass House 11 Riverside Drive, Dundee DD1 4NY, www.sssc.uk.com
    Wales: Care Council for Wales, Southgate House Wood Street, Cardiff CF10 1EW, www.socialcare.wales
    Northern Ireland Social Care Council, 19-25 Great Victoria St, Belfast BT2 7AQ, www.niscc.info
    & 4th Floor, James House, 2 Cromac Avenue, Belfast, BT7 2JA

Moving & Handling of People in Care Settings

Health and Safety Executive, Redgrave Court, Merton Road, Bootle, Merseyside, L20 7HS, *www.hse.gov.uk*
Health Service Ombudsman,11th Floor, Millbank Towers Millbank, London SW1P, *www.ombudsman.org.uk*
    Scotland, Bridgeside House 99 McDonald Road, Edinburgh EH7 4NS, *www.spso.org.uk*
    Wales: 1 Ffordd yr Hen Gae, Pencoed CF35 5LJ, *www.ombudsman.wales*
Muscular Dystrophy Campaign, 7-11 Prescott Place, London, SW4 6BS *www.muscular-dystrophy.org*
National Association of Care & Support Workers, International House, 24 Holborn Viaduct, London Ec1A 2BN, www.*nacas.org.uk*
National Back Exchange, Linden Barns, Greens Norton Road, Towcester NN12 8AW, *www.nationalbackexchange.org*
National Back Pain Association, 16 Elmtree Road Teddington, Middlesex TW11 SST
National Osteoporosis Society, Camerton, Bath, BA2 0PJ, *www.nos.org.uk*
Spinal Injuries Association, 76 St James's Lane, London, N10 3DF, *www.spinal.co.uk*
The Law Society, 50 Chancery Lane, London, WC2A 1SX, *www.lawsociety.org.uk*

Moving and handling and certified first aid training service provider:

TPS, First Aid Certification, Halkevi Centre, 31-33 Dalston Lane, London E8 3DF, *www.theprotectionservice.org*
AMBA, Holistic Moving and Handling Training Consultants
info@ambaconsultltd.com
www.ambaconsultltd.com

Care Service Provider
Supreme Care Services Limited, 9 Crown Parade, Crown Lane, Morden, Surrey, SM4 5DA, *www.supremecare.co.uk*

Indexes

back injury, 80, 117
Care Act, *8, 17, 40, 48, 153*
Care plan, *41, 42*
Care Plan
   handling plan, 26, 27, 41, 42, 50, 61, 102, 103
Children and young persons, *83*
Compliance, *1, 13, 17, 41, 53*
Consent, *10, 48*
Duty of care, *41, 141*
   legal obligation, *25, 41*
Ergonomic risk assessment process. *See* Risk Assessment
First Aid, *51, 80, 145*
Fluids and nutrition. *See* nutrition
GDPR, *8, 51, 52, 153*
hoist, *20, 21, 44, 46, 108, 109, 122, 125, 126, 127, 129, 130, 131*
   Hoisting, *109, 126, 127, 128, 130, 131*
   Hoisting checklist, *128*
Holistic Approach, *53*
   Code of Conduct, *41, 54, 55, 56, 57, 87*
   Communication, *44, 58, 60*
   Confidentiality, *61, 62*
   COSHH, *8, 66, 153*
   Emergency procedures in the workplace, *67*
   Equality & diversity, *58*
   Holistic Care, *55, 59, 70*
   Infections, *65*
   nutrition, *17, 64, 137, 143*
   Safeguarding, *41, 63, 83, 144, 151*
   Values, *58*
HSWA, *8, 37, 153*
Human back
   Biomechanics, *71*
   MSDs, *31, 32, 77, 78*
   Vertebral column, *73*
Human Back, *71*
Learning disability, *84*
Legislation, *27, 30, 32, 126, 128, 141, 142*
Lifting activity
   activity, *13, 20, 30, 31, 34, 43, 44, 47, 48, 49, 51, 55, 58, 61, 72, 81, 83, 87, 88, 89, 90, 95, 102, 103, 106, 108, 111, 124, 125, 126*
Lifting equipment, *21*
Lifting operation. *See* Lifting activity
Load, *22, 45, 75, 96*
LOLER, *8, 15, 22, 34, 35, 99, 119, 126, 139, 153*
Manual handling, *22, 30, 31, 58, 77, 88, 90, 96, 152*
Mental Capacity, *48, 49, 153*
   MCA, *48, 49, 50, 82, 84*
MHOR, *8, 22, 30, 31, 32, 33, 53, 54, 88, 89, 94, 127, 137, 138, 139, 141, 148, 153*
MHSWR, *8, 16, 32, 35, 36, 83, 84, 94, 141, 153*
moving and handling, *13, 15, 17, 18, 19, 20, 27, 28, 30, 31, 41, 42, 43, 46, 47, 48, 49, 50, 51, 53, 54, 58, 60, 61, 64, 65, 66, 81, 82, 83, 85, 101, 102, 103, 107, 110, 111, 128, 136, 137, 139, 140, 141, 144, 145, 154*
neck injury, 80
organisation, *10, 21, 25, 26, 28, 35, 38, 42, 43, 47, 51, 62, 68, 85, 89, 98, 99, 100, 103, 111, 139, 140, 145*

Organisations, *21, 28, 29, 34, 43, 52, 146, 154*
paraplegia, *79*
Personal Care, *110*
Physical Illnesses, *81*
Policy and procedure, *43*
PUWER, *9, 15, 35, 36, 99, 119, 139, 153*
quadriplegia, *79*
Research, 137
RIDDOR, *9, 36, 38, 39, 41, 62, 102, 138, 141, 153*
Risk Assessment, *9, 45, 94, 95, 96, 127*
   MAC tool, *94*
   RAPP tool, *95*
Significant Others, *11, 25, 28, 51*
Spinal cord, *74, 78*
spinal cord injuries, *79*
Statistics, 8, *23*, 152
Strategy for handling people, *103*
tetraplegia, *79*

Trainers, *28, 139*
Training, *1, 8, 13, 17, 28, 40, 62, 127, 136, 140, 141, 142, 143, 146*
   induction, 18, *28, 43, 55, 62, 136, 140, 141*, 145
   Knowledge, *53, 136*
   refresher, 18, *28, 62*, 137, 140
   skills, *8, 10, 11, 20, 29, 37, 44, 48, 54, 58, 60, 68, 85, 100, 136, 137, 140, 141, 143, 144*
   understanding, *19, 20, 46, 48, 54, 58, 84, 100, 136, 137, 141*
   unsafe, *19, 30, 31, 111, 112, 113, 116*
   Bear Hug, *112*
   Blanket Lift, *115*, 116
   Drag Lift, *112*
   Orthodox Lift, *116*
   Pivot, 114
Unsafe lifting techniques. *See* Unsafe

Printed in Great Britain
by Amazon

41548271R00091